# PARASITES
# AND
# SKIN DISEASES

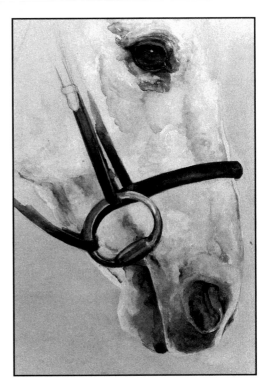

# PARASITES
# AND
# SKIN DISEASES

Peter Gray

MVB, MRCVS

J. A. Allen
London

British Library Cataloguing in Publication Data
A catalogue record for this book is available from the British Library

ISBN 0-85131-624-7

Published in Great Britain in 1995 by
J. A. Allen & Company Limited
1 Lower Grosvenor Place
London SW1W 0EL

Production editor: Bill Ireson
Illustrator: Maggie Raynor
Cover designer: Nancy Lawrence
Printed in Hong Kong

*To the memory of*
*Molly*
*whose 93 years were eminently worthwhile*

## 8 Bacterial and Fungal Diseases  141

## 9 Allergies and Poisons  154

## 10 Tumours and Other Conditions  167

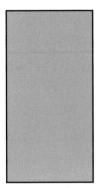

# Acknowledgements

I would like to express my gratitude to Professor Brian J. Sheahan, MA, MVB, MS, PhD, MRCVS, MRCPath, of the Department of Veterinary Pathology, University College Dublin, for the photograhic material he has so generously provided and for his help in reading the manuscript.

My thanks also to a number of individuals: Professor Kenneth P. Baker, MA, MSc, Phd, DVD, FRCVS, of the Department of Veterinary Clinical Medicine, University College Dublin, for his help with that part of the book on skin diseases; David Byron, of MSD AGVET, for his most generous help with material, especially the use of the many photographs included in the text; Jane Parry, BVetMed, MRCVS, also of MSD AGVET, for reference material she supplied; Jacqueline Meldon, of Pfizer Animal Health Limited, who also very kindly provided photographic material; and Deborah J. Baker, BVetMed., MRCVS, of Hoechst UK Limited.

To Raymond Hopes, BVMS, MRCVS, of Rossdale and Partners, Newmarket, Suffolk, I am indebted for the use of photographs and slides on skin conditions. For the photographs they supplied, my thanks to: Peter D. Rossdale, MA, PhD, DESM, FRCVS; Colin K. Peace, MA, VetMB, MRCVS; and Alan Wright, BVSc, MRCVS.

For help provided I would also like to thank: Roger R. Dawson, BSc, PhD, Animal Medicines Training Regulatory Authority (AMTRA); Roger Cook, National Office of Animal Health (NOAH); and the staff of the Wellcome Library, Royal College of Veterinary Surgeons (RCVS).

My special thanks, too, to Maggie Raynor for her excellent artwork; to Bill Ireson for his production editing; to Nancy Lawrence for the cover design; and to my publishers for their help and encouragement.

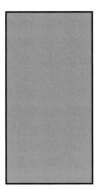 # Illustration Acknowledgements

I am grateful to the individuals and organisations listed below for giving their permission to reproduce original material. Each subject used is listed by the relevant page number in this book.

Note that many subjects have been enlarged or reduced and are therefore *not to scale*.

J. A. Allen & Co. Ltd.: p. 31, p. 93.
Raymond Hopes: p. 101 (bottom), p. 135, p. 159 (two), p. 172 (two), p. 181, p. 186, p. 188, p. 190, p. 191.
MSD AGVET: p. 24 (two), p. 26, p. 30, p. 36, p. 40 (top), p. 43 (top), p. 46, p. 51 (two), p. 58 (top and centre), p. 63, p. 114, p. 120 (two), p. 124 (three), p. 130 (bottom), p. 134 (top), p. 139 (two).
Colin K. Peace: p. 100 (two).
Pfizer Limited: p. 8, p. 43 (centre and bottom), p. 58 (bottom), p. 71.
Peter D. Rossdale: p. 176.
Brian J. Sheahan: p. 9, p. 40 (bottom), p. 169 (three).
Alan Wright: p. 130 (top), p. 134 (bottom), p. 150 (two), p. 171.

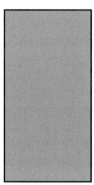

# Introduction

Parasites and skin diseases of horses are two subjects about which the average horse owner knows little. The difficulty lies in that they are specialist subjects, filled with their own technical terminology and therefore hard to interpret.

However, the clinical importance of these fields is evident in everday horse management. Worms and other parasites have a significant ongoing effect on growth and production. Skin conditions, be they contagious or not, are a familiar form of equine disease and a regular reason why horses cannot be ridden.

In attempting to make these subjects understandable to the lay person, therefore, it is necessary in this book to begin at the practical base. For example, common names, like 'redworm' and 'lungworm', are used in conjunction with the generic names, *Strongylus* and *Dictyocaulus*. For correctness, however, the generic names will be used in parentheses in section headings, but every effort is made to enable the reader to gain the information he or she requires without being overcome by the technical nomenclature which is vital to the scientist/veterinarian.

Similarly, in discussing the effects of parasite infection, it is not intended to delve into the complexities of equine pathology. Yet it should be understood that pathology means the study of diseases, or, more properly, the study of the changes in body tissues that result from disease. Thus, a worm is not just an undesirable resident of the digestive system; it may damage the lining to the bowel, it may migrate through other tissues, causing damage to remote organs. It may also interfere with digestion, preventing the absorption of food elements from the bowel; this may lead to weight loss, stunted growth, and improper development of the horse's skeleton. Pathology therefore is a vital part of our discourse here; anyone who has an interest in horses and responsibility for their welfare will be better for an understanding of pathology, and more able to understand the wider practical effects of a given disease.

This book is, then, organised in a way that should make most sense to such a reader. It is not the way in which parasites and skin diseases are dealt with in professional literature, but that need not be of concern. Any reader who digests the contents of this book and wants more information might well be ready to tackle the complexities of specialist professional texts. In order to help the reader with the more technical terms, a glossary is included at the end of the book.

A parasite is a living organism that lives upon or within another living organism from whence it ekes its existence. Its affect on the host varies but may occur directly through invasion of tissues, or through the ingestion of blood as the redworm does. Mange mites live on surface cells, some even burrowing within the skin. Some parasites live within the bowel, in the lumen (centre of the tract) unattached, obtaining their food from the bowel contents.

Parasites that exist within the animal are called endoparasites. Those that live on the skin are called ectoparasites.

The animal that supports the parasite is referred to as the host. In this book, the host in all cases is the horse and we will at times distinguish between the influence parasites have on horses at different stages of growth.

In the main we are dealing with helminth parasites among which are the common worms (divided into nematodes, cestodes and trematodes) of the horse's bowel and arthropod parasites (ticks, mites, lice and flies).

Many parasites are what is known as 'host-specific', meaning they confine themselves to a single species. Others are not and can be found in different animals. It is evident that a worm which is common to cattle, sheep and horses would therefore have a special significance where each of these species were grazed on the same piece of land.

Each parasite has a specific location within a host where it is most commonly found – called a predilection site – and which may play a part in the technical naming of the parasite. Needless to say parasitic infestation may cause interference with the horse's body defences and thus pave the way for secondary infection with bacteria and viruses. A further problem (associated mainly with ectoparasites) is the ability of some parasites to transmit disease (e.g. encephalitis virus and swamp fever, transmitted by biting flies and mosquitoes; human malaria is a protozoan disease, transmitted by mosquitoes).

Other factors which may influence disease are the age of the host and physical condition, also matters like season, climate, geographic location, and so on. Internal worm burdens have a more insidious effect in cold, wet conditions and external parasites may irritate most in warmer weather.

Climatic factors also dictate the manner in which parasites survive outside the host. Most endoparasites lay eggs which pass onto pasture in the faeces. These may hatch into larvae which are ingested by the next host. The capacity of larvae to survive externally is influenced by heat and cold, the quality of the pasture, exposure to sunlight, and so on. Because of this life cycle, horses which are stabled are less likely to encounter parasites than when kept at grass. However, parasitic risk is not completely eliminated by stabling, and stable hygiene is important in preventing spread of disease.

Of course, very few infections are caused by a single parasite. The type and number involved may vary, and there may be external and internal parasites occurring at the same time. This, naturally, will influence the effect on the host. The most important aspect of all this is the daily influence parasites have on management. What are the risks of your horse being affected by diseases which are not altogether evident on the surface? How can you recognise a worm infection? What is the life cycle? What is the prevention? What is the treatment?

Horses, being animals which are kept for pleasure, not food, suffer because research on their diseases is often deemed uneconomical. We must rely therefore to some extent on information from other sources, like research into cattle and sheep diseases. Yet this does not reduce the value of the information as long as it is understood that principles applying to parasitic infection in general may be diluted in certain circumstances because of the nature of the horse. The horse owner is, of course, more interested in bone development, or diseases of bone that may ensue from nutritional problems. He or she is also interested in weight gain, in the full, normal physical development of an athletic animal; of its ability to perform, to stand up to training and to carry weight. But our primary interest must be in the soundness of our horses, not weight gain *per se*. We simply wish for the animal to reach its natural potential without due hindrance.

Skin diseases are also complex and have a variety of causes besides external parasites. For example, modern medicine recognises such diverse causes as infection, diet, contact with irritant or allergenic substances, allergies, hereditary and auto-immune disease. Each of these are dealt with in some detail in this book, hopefully thus making it easier for the reader to understand and recognise the different expressions of skin disease. There is a great deal that horse owners themselves can do to minimise the problems related to them.

In a book combining these two subjects, parasites and skin diseases, it is inevitable that there might be some duplication or variation from an ideal line. For example, the botfly parasitises the horse's stomach in its larval stages; the warble fly, when it affects horses, is most significant when a developing larva appears under the skin of the back. In this book, both are included with other conditions caused by flies, and are therefore treated as external parasites. The reader should not suffer on that account.

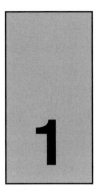

# 1 The Effects of Infestation

In any parasitic infection, the effect of the parasite (pathology) depends on a number of factors. The nature of the parasite and the way it lives is critical to this. In other words, coughing caused by lungworms is a reflection of the presence of the worm *Dictyocaulus arnfieldi* in the air passages (trachea and bronchi) and the irritation it causes there. Yet it is known that large numbers of the same worm can exist, for example, in the donkey's air passages with little clinical effect. This is not abnormal and simply indicates the influence of a parasite on different hosts.

Parasitic diseases are divided into those which infect animals internally and those that infest the skin and appendages.

Factors affecting pathology are discussed below.

## Host Specificity

Many parasites are host-specific (they set up disease only in a specific host). However, the same parasites may exist (without causing any, or an equivalent, disease) in other species of animals (as with lungworm) or may be incapable of living their life cycles outside their natural host. The equine lungworm is peculiar in that the horse is not the natural host, and consequently the worm usually fails to complete its life cycle while still causing clinical disease in the horse. The problem here is often with diagnosis, which is dependent on the detection of immature worm types (larvae) in the faeces. Negative results do not eliminate lungworm (because the worms may fail to fully mature and reproduce in the horse) and very often only treatment with an effective drug will rule out their presence.

| *Adult worms are found in the following sites* | Digestive system, including the oesophagus<br>Liver<br>Lungs, bronchi and trachea<br>Ligamentum nuchae<br>Peritoneum<br>Eye |
|---|---|

| *Immature worms are found in the following sites* | Digestive system<br>Blood vascular system (especially in arteries to bowel)<br>Liver<br>Lungs<br>Tongue<br>Brain and spinal cord<br>Kidneys |
|---|---|

Similarly, the liver fluke, *Fasciola*, can infect horses grazing ground contaminated by cattle or sheep. The fluke can enter the liver and cause symptoms (for example, anaemia and jaundice) although there are often no fluke eggs in the faeces. Treatment is carried out as part of an elimination process therefore and the diagnosis is only confirmed by an improvement in the health of the horse thereafter – hardly evidence that would satisfy a scientist. Liver fluke is not a very common condition of horses in the UK, though it does occur; it is more common in Ireland where climatic factors favour the habitat of the snail intermediate host. These examples should be a warning, however, as to what can be expected from parasitic disease.

# Quantity of Parasite

Quantity is a critical factor in infection as, inevitably, the more parasites involved the more serious the effect they will have on the host. The concentration of worms available to any animal is a matter for management control and is greatly influenced by poor management practices that allow infection to build up.

# Endoparasites in Disease

How endoparasites cause disease depends on a number of factors. Those of importance are: the manner in which the parasite lives and feeds; its predilection site; whether or not it causes tissue damage; if it migrates through body organs. Some worms, like the mature roundworm, *Parascaris equorum*, living free within the small intestine, may get so large and be present in such numbers as to physically block the bowel, a particular problem in young foals. Yet the mature worm does little harm to the bowel itself, although larval stages migrate through body tissues and reach the bowel by way of the lungs. While there may be no external signs of these stages, there is no doubt that such tissue meanderings have a significance, not least in the discomfort and pain they must cause the host. Large numbers of immature worms may pass through organs like the lungs and liver in heavy infestations; this is clear from the traces they leave which are seen later, on post-mortem examination. It is not inconceivable that such meanderings could precipitate overt respiratory disease, especially in young animals; yet the suspicion may not arise at the time, the symptoms being attributed to the secondary effect of bacteria and viruses. The possible allergic effects of this could also play a clinical part, because tissue reactions that result from previous exposure to a parasite can further enhance the disease process. A sensitised animal (one that has had previous contact with a parasite) reacts in a way that could mean local tissue swelling, fluid effusion, increased blood flow to the part; all of which, in an area like the lung, could further inhibit respiration.

It is also thought possible that fluke infection lowers resistance to some gut parasites.

## Specific Effects of Endoparasites

The effects of infection are manifested in many ways. Some are discussed below.

### Physical Injury

Damage to tissues occurs, firstly, by the effect of mature worms that live off the surface of the bowel. These, most notably the large redworms (strongyles), attach to the bowel lining and may even tear away large plugs of tissue which they digest. The larval stages of these worms also cause injury to the lining of blood vessels through which they travel.

Immature stages of small redworms develop within the surface of the bowel, thereby causing local tissue damage, often forming nodules, and resulting in ulcerated areas or more general inflammation (enteritis).

Physical injury to more remote tissues occurs as a result of larvae migrating through organs (for example, liver and lungs, as already mentioned). This results in local tissue destruction which is followed by repair through the medium of scar tissue.

## Mechanical Obstruction

The horse roundworm, *Parascaris*, also the large tapeworm, *Anoplocephala,* can cause mechanical obstruction of the bowel. *Parascaris* worms may also block the bile ducts, resulting in jaundice.

## Food Deprivation

Parasites such as *Parascaris* and *Anoplocephala* may compete with the host for ingested food. Growth of the animal is therefore affected because of lost nutrients.

## Anorexia

Anorexia (the voluntary reduction of food intake) is a clinical result of some worm diseases, the animal thus losing weight because of reduced food intake. It has been shown that where appetite is not affected (i.e. the animal is not anorexic) in this way weight loss is less severe.

The cause of anorexia is not always clear. It is possibly due to an effect on nerve endings in the bowel, thus affecting appetite by direct influence on the brain. It is also possibly due to pain or to disturbances in metabolism as a result of a worm burden. A factor in this may be altered acidity of bowel contents. It may also occur in response to a failure of digestion

*Horse roundworm: physical size of worm may obstruct the bowel in foals*

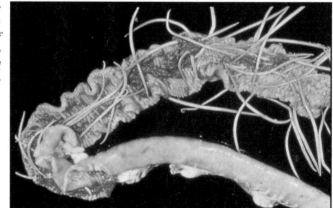

that leaves undigested material in the stomach and bowel; or any change in the number or type of bacteria in the gut could affect amino acid production – thus affecting appetite.

Anorexia is a known side-effect of fluke infestation in cattle and sheep, in coccidiosis, and in other non-specified parasitic infections. It is a recognised effect of some worm infestations of horses.

## Absorption of Food

The process of digestion includes absorption of food constituents into the circulation from the bowel. Such absorption is adversely influenced by direct injury to the lining of the bowel, preventing normal transfer of substances like proteins, fats and minerals. This further complicates the clinical picture, because undigested food passes along the bowel and may putrify, resulting in possible constipation or diarrhoea as well as anorexia.

Failure of digestion may result in the breakdown and use of body tissues (for example, muscle protein) to maintain life and this may be exacerbated by the physical loss of blood proteins into the bowel as a result of tissue reactions and haemorrhage.

Parasitic infection increases the amount of protein in the gut not only because of interference with normal digestion (preventing protein absorption) but because there is loss of protein from the blood (due to blood-sucking and tissue tearing) and also, as already mentioned, because of serum and plasma entering the bowel as a result of tissue injury. This varies with the specific parasite and with the level of infection.

Even when this protein is broken down and reabsorbed later in the digestive process, energy is used, thus further depleting body reserves. Proteins that are not digested pass into the large bowel where they may

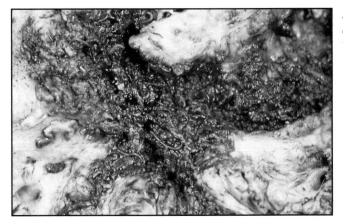

*Large redworm larvae in a blood vessel wall*

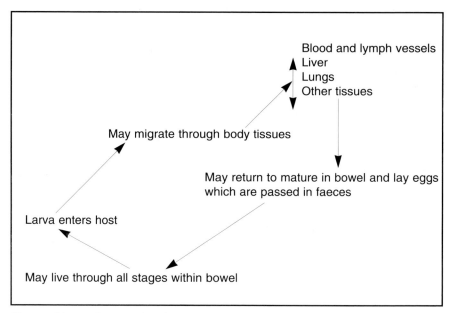

*Nature of internal worm migrations*

be broken down and the constituent amino acids used by bacteria. If not degraded, they are excreted in faeces and thus adversely affect the nitrogen balance of the host.

## Anaemia

Anaemia occurs as a result of blood loss; this can be caused by blood-sucking parasites. It can also be a result of haemorrhage from damaged areas of bowel or from failure of synthesis resulting from dietary problems like faulty absorption. Into this scenario comes malnutrition, which can be exacerbated by anorexia and plasma leakage; and also competition between host and parasite for food constituents which are either ingested or synthesised by the host.

Some parasites possess anti-clotting agents which allow bleeding to continue even after they have moved on to new sites. Adult large strongyles ingest sizeable plugs of bowel lining, thus causing severe damage to the bowel, allowing bleeding and leading to ulceration.

Anaemia is a feature of redworm infestation, but it is also an observed clinical sign of fluke infestation. Anaemia with fluke occurs because of whole blood ingestion by fluke and also haemolysis (destruction of red blood cells) - possibly due to toxin production.

*Symptoms of infection*

Anaemia
Constipation and diarrhoea
Poor coat
Pot belly
Weight loss

Vitamin levels are lowered in some parasitic infections. The production of anaemia where there is no direct bleeding could thus be explained (e.g. vitamin B12 is involved in blood metabolism). Anaemia can also occur due to haemolysis, as in trypanosomiasis, or schistosomiasis (protozoan diseases).

Sheep with haemonchosis (a roundworm) may have to replace all circulating red cells every three weeks, as opposed to a normal of every four months. Such an effect in the horse would be obviously serious for competing animals.

## Bowel Damage

Damage to the lining of the bowel may further complicate matters by reducing the secretion of essential digestive enzymes.

Parasitic infection possibly has no effect on calcium absorption (although there are many non-parasitic situations in which calcium absorption is less than ideal) but has been shown to reduce phosphorus. This may explain faulty skeletal development in some infections.

## Obstruction

*Parascaris* infection of the foal is capable of obstructing the lumen, and of increasing the diameter of the small intestine; the degree being related to the number of parasites present. This could extend to a point where the bowel was ruptured.

Worm burdens are also known to increase the weight of the small intestine. This probably reflects altered digestive processes as well as an

*Affect of worms within bowel*

Allergic tissue reactions
Anorexia
Blockage or distension
Blood and serum loss
Digestive disturbances
Direct tissue damage
Pain

increase in water content of the digesta. Gut inflammation may increase motility of the bowel and thus reduce absorption by moving contents on before they have time to be digested; conversely, there is a known reduction of colonic activity in ponies with strongylosis, a possible cause of constipation.

## Allergic Reactions

The interaction that occurs between host and parasite results in allergic reactions. Such reactions may further complicate the nature of disease, especially where there is a gradual intake of worms, allowing time for development of these immune-related reactions. It is believed that the enzyme phospholipase in the small intestine and the production of eosinophils (a type of white blood cell, thought to be the source of the phospholipase) in bone marrow are associated with the development of immunity and expulsion of parasites. Gamma globulins increase in the blood as infection continues, representing part of the same immune process.

Immunity develops as a result of exposure to infection. Young animals are therefore more susceptible (having no acquired immunity), showing more severe symptoms and having a higher mortality rate. While some older animals may rid themselves of parasites by a mechanism known as self-cure, and remain vitually parasite free, others do not. Considering this, it is necessary to treat adult horses on a regular basis in order to limit environmental contamination for younger animals.

With initial parasite infections, therefore, only physical destruction of tissues occurs (with bleeding and scar formation), while gradually, with continued worm intake, allergic reactions occur and may add to the adverse clinical effect. The parasites cause acute local pathology which greatly exacerbates the disease process.

Immunity, when it develops, is marked by lowered faecal egg counts to virtually zero. Adult worm counts in the horse fall significantly and remain low, generally, throughout life. It should be appreciated, however, that immunity in worm infestations is not a simple matter and scientists are constantly in search of vaccines which may help to eliminate specific worm problems.

And it is much simpler to produce vaccines against bacteria and viruses.

## Pain

Pain is a considered symptom of worm infection, the effect of which can be to suppress appetite and further exacerbate disease. Pain may be significant in acute infections of foals and is possibly caused by tissue destruction, the accumulation of fluid, and physical distension of the bowel.

## Oedema

Dependent oedema and accumulation of fluid in the abdominal cavity (ascites) may contribute to the pot-bellied appearance of foals affected with worms. This is a result of malnutrition and disturbance in metabolism and body fluid balance – the cumulative effect of parasitism.

## Diarrhoea

Another effect/symptom of worm infestation, diarrhoea in itself contributes to dehydration and weight loss. It is caused by a number of the problems already listed and also includes failure of digestion, putrefaction of the digesta and damage to the bowel lining.

Constipation may also be a feature and increase the prospect of colic (an aspect of strongyle infection of horses at almost any age).

## Aneurysms

There is a stage when the burden of worms may be too little to cause external disease signs, although with redworms in particular, there may be serious lesions developing within blood vessels as the immature, larval stages migrate. The consequence of this may be the formation of aneurysms (a dilatation of the blood vessel wall) with the consequent risk of emboli (in this case a plug of immature worms carried from a large to a smaller blood vessel, thus causing a blockage), perhaps leading to death of the host through colic, haemorrhage, and so on.

# Signs of Infestation

The external signs of worm infestation are often obscure or so general as to give no specific evidence of the underlying cause (for example, loss of weight, retarded development, anaemia, poor coat). With increasing worm numbers, health (as indicated by appetite, weight, development) suffers and the host veers from a state of clinical normality to one of disease. It is therefore critical that we have methods for diagnosis, control and treatment. A full understanding of the nature, habits and propagation of parasites is essential to this.

In any outbreak, only a number of horses in a herd will show signs of disease. The result of the infection, however, may lower, for example, productivity; reproduction may be similarly affected. Other horses will also probably be affected by disease but with symptoms which are less marked.

## Management of Infestation

The number of worms ingested at any one time is critical to disease; the larger the dose and the greater the frequency of ingestion, the more severe are the signs. Dosage is something over which we have some control as long as we understand the way in which grazing land becomes infected and the factors influencing it (for example, environmental, or where in addition to horses other species are grazing the land). We can immediately reduce the dosage by moving affected horses to clean pasture. However, should we allow a carry-over of infection (by failing to treat the horses being moved), the clean pasture will soon also be infected.

Age is relevant to disease – because young animals are generally more susceptible than old. An adult may have an acquired immunity or a natural age resistance to infection; so it is important to consider this in dealing with both young and old horses. However it would be a mistake to imagine that older horses do not pose a threat to younger animals, or that they have no need to be wormed.

Poor nutrition will also affect disease. Those animals on low-protein diets are less well able to resist infection than those on a higher plane of nutrition.

Body weight is affected by infections of the bowel, and also by infection of the liver, kidneys, and the circulatory and respiratory systems. Roundworms are the parasites most commonly involved, but infections with tapeworms or fluke may also depress growth or weight. Although worm-free horses on bad diets may appear to have worms because of their lack of condition, they will also be more seriously affected by worms when the quality of their feed is inadequate. It is proven that parasitised animals thrive better when moved to fresh pasture of equal nutritional quality, but which is worm free.

## Climatic Conditions

Season and climate are of prime importance as most parasites favour warmth and moisture during their external development stages. Eggs hatch more readily and larvae develop faster on lush pasture, in warm, humid conditions. A greater number of larvae survive in summer than winter months (although bright sunshine kills off larvae in southern latitudes) and some infestations are more serious in dry weather and on poor quality pasture. This is not to say that direct sunshine won't kill exposed larvae in northern latitudes, but warmer conditions, especially with added humidity, will favour parasitic development whereas cold winter weather is more likely to kill eggs and larvae which are exposed. Some survive winter conditions due to the toughness of their eggs or particular larval stages.

Weather is also critical, of course, to the ability of a host to survive

---

**Spring**

- Surviving eggs and larvae on pasture
- Encysted small strongyles emerge and mature in bowel
- Migrating large strongyles emerge and mature in bowel
- Bots leave the host

*Mild weather favours pasture larval development. Worm burdens in adults lead to carry over of infection for young animals on clean pasture (e.g. emerging large and small strongyles)*

**Summer**

- Increasing pasture contamination
- Heavy burdens in untreated animals
- Intensive grazing produces 'rough' and 'lawn' areas in paddocks
- Bot and other flies on wing

*Strong sunshine destroys exposed larvae. Wet, humid weather favours larval development*

**Autumn**

- Mature worms lay fewer eggs
- Heavy frosts reduce larval numbers, killing off bots and other flies

*Cold weather kills most eggs and larvae*

**Winter**

- Stabled or barn-kept horses may be infected with *Oxyuris*, *Parascaris*, *Strongyloides*, liver fluke, tapeworm

*But* Parascaris *eggs,* Trichostrongylus *and* Cyathostomum *larvae are resistant to cold*

---

*Seasonal influences*

infection and it is recognised that more parasitised animals die in adverse weather conditions.

## Mixed Infection

Awareness of the consequences of mixed infection is, too, a matter of importance. Under natural field conditions, mixed infections are the rule, and the added burden of different species of parasite makes the disease consequences more significant. Sometimes, however, mixed infections may create competition between parasites which favour the host.

## Reproduction and Lactation

Impaired physical development may delay puberty in young animals, a natural consequence of parasitic infestation.

From comparisons with other species, fluke may reduce reproductive efficiency in horses by affecting the general state of health. This can lead to infertility, possibly resulting from lowered uterine disease resistance and poor follicle development in the ovaries. There may also be impaired milk production, and increased early embryonic death. There could also be a reduction in colostrum and milk quality, possibly resulting in increased disease susceptibility and unthriftiness in foals.

## Productivity

Interference with body calcium and phosphorus levels is likely to affect normal bone development in young horses as in other species: for example, osteoporosis and osteomalacia have been detected in lambs suffering from particular worm infestations. Bone length and volume may suffer and epiphyseal growth may be affected.

Protein metabolism is critical to normal physical development, and has a particular relevance to muscle formation. The fact that absorption of proteins is reduced in worm infestations is therefore of prime consideration in horse growth and development, a critical problem for young, developing, athletic animals. It may even occur that existing body proteins have to be broken down in order to sustain life, thus further exacerbating the problems caused by disease. Muscle growth is therefore inhibited as well as skeletal growth, and muscle development is further inhibited by lowered rates of activity caused by weakness and malnutrition. The liver in these cases comes under pressure to produce more protein because of the shortfall, and the materials for this increase must come from existing body resources when the horse's digestive intake is inadequate, or when there is uncontrolled loss. Such a sequence of events can further affect skeletal growth, lactation and reproduction. It may also influence red blood cell manufacture, causing anaemia.

## Ectoparasites

The effect of ectoparasites usually depends on the size of the invading population and on the state of nutrition. High numbers of ectoparasites may be the result of ill-health, not the cause of it. In some species of animals, ectoparasites are known to reduce milk and egg production, also wool growth.

Anaemia may be due to blood sucking lice. Flies, too, can cause 'worry' in horses and may also act as the intermediate hosts or mechanical carriers of disease.

However, more of this later. We now need to look at endoparasites in more detail.

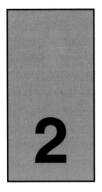

# 2 Internal Parasites

The internal parasites of the horse are confined to five main biological groupings: namely *Nematoda*, *Cestoda*, *Trematoda*, *Protozoa*, and *Insecta*. The commonly known worms of horses, roundworms, tapeworms and fluke fall into the first three of these groupings, respectively; in the last two groupings, *Coccidia* are an example of a protozoan species and bots and warbles are internal parasites belonging to *Insecta*.

Much of this chapter is concerned with nematodes. We start with the most common of them, the roundworm, as they are by far the most important group of internal parasites in the horse.

## Roundworms (Nematodes)

Nematodes are roundworms. Their importance is due not only in their availability and clinical effect but also economically.

Like the common earthworm, nematodes are elongated and taper at both ends. They have a digestive tract and mouthparts which, as in the large strongyles (possessing teeth), are often adapted for feeding on the host. Nematodes also have a tough skin. Males are smaller than females with which they mate; the minute anatomical differences that occur between individual species are critical factors in classification.

However, these are matters of academic interest and will only be referred to in passing here where this is deemed important. The most significant roundworms, clinically, are the large and small strongyles, ascarids and *Oxyuris* (pinworm).

Roundworms are sufficiently numerous to be a constant ongoing problem and their importance is often overlooked because their everyday influence is not always readily apparent. Many roundworms have a direct life cycle (no intermediate host involved) in which the adult worm matures in the bowel (or in the bronchi in the case of lungworm) and the females lay thousands of eggs that pass out in the faeces; these then develop through several stages until they gain the capacity to infect other horses, sometimes as eggs containing larvae but mostly as larvae, known as 'infective larvae'.

If environmental conditions are favourable, excreted eggs develop to the infective stage in a short space of time; these are then capable of maturing within a new host and so continuing the cycle. Hatched larvae thrive on pastures, though they are harmed by extreme cold or direct sunlight. When they become infective, larvae reside near the ground at the base of grass stems during the night. In the morning, warmed by early

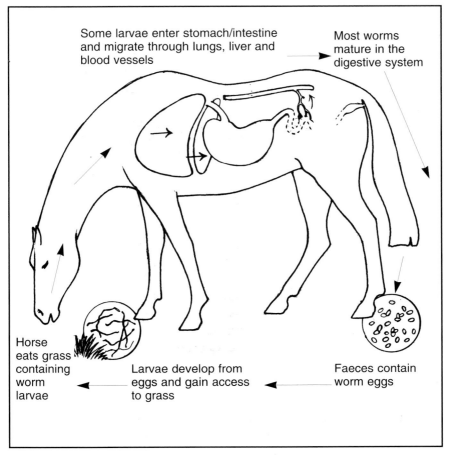

*Life-cycle of typical roundworm*

sunlight, they migrate upwards and settle near the top of the grass blades, often becoming concentrated in drops of dew. Here they are eaten by their prospective host. When ingested they either develop at their predeliction site and mature there or can, depending on species, migrate through body tissues and organs before reaching it.

There are individual variations within this format. In some cases, e.g. that of *Parascaris*, the horse eats eggs containing second stage larvae. These mature in the gut and penetrate through the gut wall thus gaining access to systemic tissues. They travel to the lungs where they make their way into the airways and climb the trachea, there to be swallowed and to eventually mature to egg-laying adults in the bowel. *Strongyloides* (the threadworm), on the other hand, produces larvae which can penetrate the skin, but only adult females of this species are parasitic.

*Strongyloides* larvae are capable of lung migration, which, while not seen as being of great clinical significance, could easily bear an influence on intercurrent bacterial or viral disease and, if there are significant numbers, limit respiration in animals expected to perform maximally. Adult females mature in the small intestine where they lay eggs that do not require fertilisation to develop. These eggs passed in the horse's faeces develop in the typical manner of most roundworms.

However, under ideal climatic conditions, *Strongyloides* larvae may grow into adult worms which can exist outside the host – which is a distinctly unusual feature.

Some nematode parasites have indirect life cycles, using intermediate hosts for stages of their development. Larvae of *Thelazia* (the eyeworm) and *Onchocerca* (which locates in the ligamentum nuchae of the neck) are ingested by specific insect hosts as they feed. They develop inside the insect and are deposited in a new horse when the insect feeds again. Eggs of *Habronema* (a stomach worm) and *Gonglyonema* (which resides in the gullet) are passed in the faeces but require an intermediate host for further development. The intermediate host of *Habronema* is a fly-maggot, that of *Gonglyonema* a dung-beetle.

## Large Redworm (*Strongylus*)

The horse acts as host to some 56 species of worms, classified as large strongyles, and it is not uncommon for anything up to 20 different species to parasitise an animal at any one time.

The best known of these are the large redworms, *Strongylus vulgaris*, *S. equinus* and *S. edentatus*. The large redworm (also called the blood-worm, its colour coming from blood it ingests) has certainly been one of the most insidious causes of disease in horses, not least because of the capacity of *S. vulgaris* to migrate through blood vessels, where it can form aneurysms. An aneurysm in this case is the dilation of an arterial wall (which inevitably weakens the structure), most commonly in the anterior mesenteric artery, resulting from the collection and clumping of larvae together. This may eventually result in rupture of the artery or, more often, the formation of emboli consisting of freed larvae and other blood elements which eventually block off smaller arteries and thus stop blood from reaching the tissues. This may result in what is termed 'embolic colic', which is very often terminal. However, it must be stressed that the typical life cycle of this worm results in larvae migrating back to, and reaching, egg-laying maturity in the bowel. But it is easy to see the complications that may arise from such a migratory cycle. The spectre of a horse with terminal colic caused by strongyles is not a pretty one and is likely to remain in the mind of anyone who has seen it (not least the vet who was helpless in dealing with the disease). However, as the quality and effectiveness of drugs has improved the part played by redworm infestation has been reduced and, thankfully, clinical crises

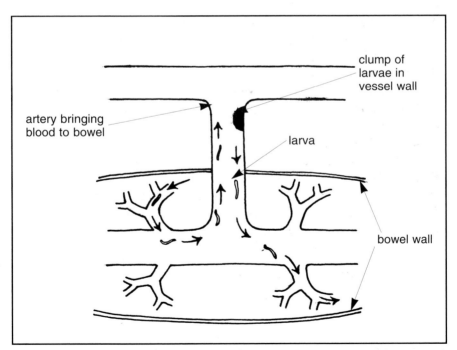

*Internal life cycle of large redworm. Larva leaves bowel and migrates through blood vessels; re-enters bowel after about four months and matures there into an egg-laying adult*

caused by this condition have become less common. Yet, management standards vary and a lack of grazing ground can mean heavy pasture contamination with worms. It would be foolish to be complacent in the use of treatment and offer any chance for redworms to dominate. There is also the danger that individuals using ill-advised dosing regimens, or patently ineffective drugs, will exacerbate problems by being unaware of the risk they run.

### Life Cycle

Adult females lay large numbers of eggs (as many as 5,000 per day) in the horse's bowel which are passed out in the faeces by which time they contain an embryo.

A first stage larva is hatched from each egg in one to two days (shorter under ideal conditions).

After feeding, this larva moults to form a second stage larva. Both of these stages exist within faeces where they live on bacteria.

Third stage larvae develop in about one week and are infective to a new host. They migrate from the faeces and contaminate soil and vegetation, from whence they are eaten.

Moisture is critical to development and in ideal conditions the infective stage can be reached in as little as three days. Infective larvae possess a protective sheath which they shed in the small intestine.

Infective larvae of *S. vulgaris* penetrate the bowel wall where they moult into fourth-stage larvae within a few days of ingestion. They then enter nearby blood vessels and wander about in the arteries for several weeks before reaching the anterior mesenteric artery, coming from the aorta, where they remain for as long as four months. After moulting to immature adults here, they return to the lumen of the large bowel, burrowing through from the blood vessels this time. Here they develop into mature egg-laying adults and eggs are laid by the new generation in about six to eight months from the initial infection.

The period from ingestion to egg-laying is called the 'prepatent period'.

There is some difference in the progress of *S. equinus* in that it migrates to the liver after moulting in the bowel wall; then it travels via other abdominal organs before maturing and laying eggs in the large bowel about nine months after infection.

Larvae of *S. edentatus* migrate to the liver before moulting and fourth stage larvae wander in the peritoneum after about nine weeks. They form nodules in the large bowel wall before entering the lumen and maturing.

The location of the mature worm is therefore the large intestine, includ-

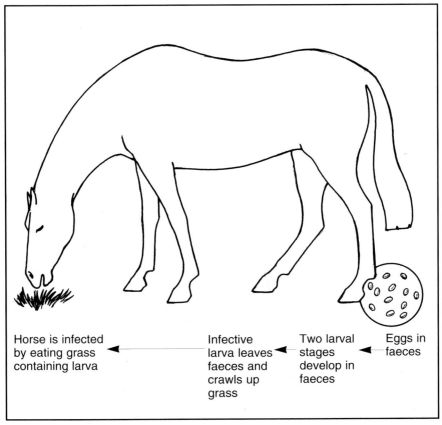

Horse is infected by eating grass containing larva ← Infective larva leaves faeces and crawls up grass ← Two larval stages develop in faeces ← Eggs in faeces

*Life cycle of redworm external to host*

ing the caecum. Redworms are universal in existence. They are of clinical significance wherever horses are kept.

**Identifying Features**

Strongyles are recognised by their distinguishing red colour. They have stout bodies that vary from 2cm to 5cm in length. *S. vulgaris* is the shortest and *S. equinus* the longest.

The mouth (buccal capsule) is well developed and armed with teeth for tearing into tissues (such as the bowel wall). Males have a copulatory bursa (shaped like grasping flaps) at the distal end for engaging with the female.

**Clinical Signs**

The most serious effect is with *S. vulgaris* in the blood vessels. The for-

*Typical redworm egg*

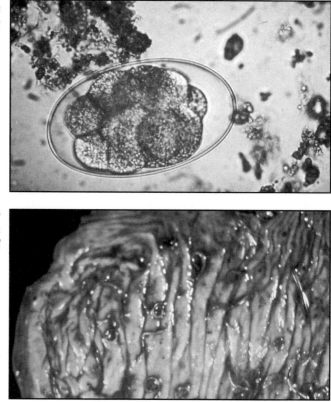

*Adult large redworms in bowel*

mation of aneurysms that contain clotted blood as well as sequestered larvae creates the unwelcome scenario of conditions such as embolic colic. There is also the possiblity that should an aneurysm rupture there will be death from sudden severe haemorrhage.

Redworms also do considerable damage to the bowel by ingesting plugs of surface material. They cause anaemia by ingesting blood as well as by creating bleeding from their feeding points. There is a resulting loss of blood protein and an associated upset in body fluid balance.

Diarrhoea may be a symptom of infection, as well as anorexia and weight loss. The immediate consequence of diarrhoea is dehydration due to fluid loss.

Liver damage and peritonitis can be caused by *S. equinus* and *S. edentatus*.

**Diagnosis**
It is difficult to confirm diagnosis of this disease before strongyle eggs are present in the faeces, although the general symptoms may suggest it.

Specific identification of individual worms depends on the location of larvae or adults, either by direct examination or by culture of faecal material. The risk of redworm infection is so great that, especially in situations where numbers of horses are kept at grass, routine preventive procedures need to be constantly in place.

**Control**
Overcrowding is likely to increase problems, and the removal of faeces from paddocks is a worthwhile part of worm control. Ploughing may be necessary where land is heavily infected. Regular faecal examination is worthwhile in monitoring the progress of this disease.

**Treatment**
Regular treatment with effective anthelmintic drugs is necessary in order to control redworms (see the next section). Adult animals need regular treatment, even where the physical condition of the animal is good, in order to lower ground contamination for younger stock.

---

- Strongyles are among the most significant worms of horses
- Migrating larvae are a common cause of serious colic
- Migrating larvae can lead to new generations of adult worms after dosing or in a new season
- Infective larvae may develop in three days from egg laying
- Females produce large numbers of eggs
- Prepatent period is six to eight months
- Larvicidal drugs are available
- Pasture hygiene is an important aspect of control

---

*Summary chart: large redworm*

# Small Redworm (including *Cyathostomum*)

There are in the region of eight different families of small strongyle and they all follow a similar type of life cycle. About 40 species of cyathostomes alone parasitise the caecum and colon of horses, and as many as 20 of these species may be found in a single infection. The small strongyles, of which the most important today is the *Cyathostomum* species, are capable of very heavy infections and counts of up to one million worms

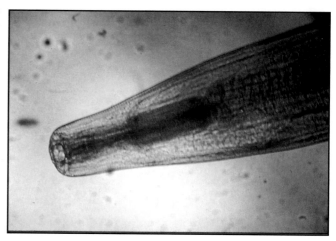

*Anterior end of small redworm. Being a 'plug feeder', this end tears out plugs of bowel wall*

have been recorded in individual animals. The worms range in size from about 5mm to 25mm in length.

## Life Cycle

The worms have a typical strongyle life cycle outside the host and go through a period of development (when they are said to be 'encysted') in the lining of the large intestine and caecum before maturing.

The prepatent period for the small redworm is shorter than for the large redworm – about five to six weeks in summer – whereas encysted larvae may remain in the wall of the bowel for as long as four months; this naturally extends the prepatent period when larvae are encysted.

## Identifying Features

Species differences are made on the basis of individual anatomy, most

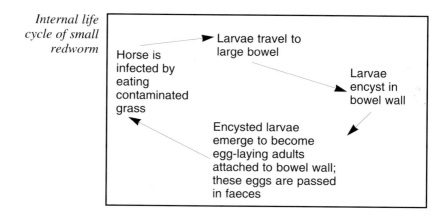

*Internal life cycle of small redworm*

Horse is infected by eating contaminated grass

Larvae travel to large bowel

Larvae encyst in bowel wall

Encysted larvae emerge to become egg-laying adults attached to bowel wall; these eggs are passed in faeces

significant of which are mouth characteristics. This type of identification is a matter for an expert and will not be detailed here.

**Clinical Signs**
In emerging from the horse's gut wall, small strongyles are responsible for a serious seasonal disease occurrence in spring. This is characterised by diarrhoea and rapid weight loss progressing to a stage of emaciation. There can be colic, also oedema of the lower abdomen. A considerable problem has been recognised with the larval stages of this worm over the years due partly to a certain level of drug resistance. However, the situation today is improving as long as a sensible routine of dosing is followed using an effective drug.

Small strongyles are a feature of mixed infection and their clinical effect is as much due to the influence of blood-sucking adults within the large intestine as the larvae in its lining. Like large strongyles, they are termed 'plug-feeders', meaning they tear away segments of bowel wall, including small blood vessels, which they digest. Being smaller, the damage caused by individual worms is less than with *Strongylus* species. However, the propensity for large infections together with drug resistance, give them a significant position as the cause of disease today.

Adult cyathostomes are also responsible for diarrhoea, weight loss and colic.

**Diagnosis**
Clinical crises caused by immature small redworms create a problem in diagnosis, as there may be few, if any, eggs found in the faeces. Small strongyle females lay about 100 eggs per day (a figure that becomes significant when there are many adult females present). Large numbers of larvae may however be found in faeces on occasion (heavy infestations) and these can then be identified.

**Control**
An essential element of control, especially where large numbers of horses are kept, is the level of pasture contamination confronting foals. Ideally mares should be treated and placed on clean pasture after foaling. However, special consideration should be given to the spring emergence of encysted larvae which may then mature and be a source of infection for foals. Efforts should be made to avoid overcrowding. Removal of faeces

from pastures is good practice – harrowing may only lead to wider pasture contamination. Selective worming with an effective drug is essential.

### Treatment

While most available anthelmintics are effective against the mature stages of redworm, proven efficacy against the tissue meandering immature larvae is restricted to ivermectin, or fenbendazole on a five-day treatment basis (also effective against encysted cyathostomes). Oxfendazole also has proven efficacy against migrating larvae. (Some species of cyathostomes have been found to be resistant to benzimidazole drugs.)

A most important time to dose for strongyles is in the spring, because at this time encysted and migrating larvae emerge to become egg-laying adults. As the new generation of strongyles is particularly fecund, it is vital they are removed before being given the opportunity to contaminate fresh pastures.

Adult large and small strongyles are susceptible to the benzimidazole group of drugs (although some small strongyles are resistant): also dichlorvos, febantel, ivermectin, levamisole, piperazine, and pyrantel pamoate (embonate). Sometimes, for greater efficacy, drugs like thiabendazole (a benzimidazole) and piperazine are used together although this practice has lost popularity due to drug resistance and the advent of more easily administered and effective drugs. Phenothiazine has also been used against large and small strongyles in the past but has been largely replaced today by more effective drugs, partly on account of toxicity.

---

- Encysted larvae are resistant to treatment
- Adult worms are resistant to some drugs
- Heavy burdens are common, leading to high pasture contamination
- Larvae are resistant in nature: may survive five months externally in cold weather
- Harrowing may expose larvae to destruction (but could spread infection)
- Mixed grazing helps reduce pasture larval counts
- Pasture hygiene is an important aspect of control
- Prepatent period varies from five weeks to four months
- Infective larvae may develop in two to three days
- Affected horses may be emaciated and scouring, especially in autumn and spring

---

*Summary chart: small redworm*

## Threadworm (*Strongyloides*)

Despite the similar name, *Strongyloides westeri* belongs to a different worm group under the nematode heading. Adult worms are most commonly encountered in suckling and weanling foals. This parasite has its peak clinical effect in the early months of life and faecal egg counts are tapering off by four to six months of age. Parasitic forms live deep in the lining of the intestine, especially the small intestine.

**Life Cycle**

*S. westeri* is unique among animal parasites in having alternate free-living and parasitic generations – in both of which five larval stages are separated by four moults. There are no parasitic males (only females) and parasitic females have no male sex organs, although they still manage to lay larva-producing eggs. These larvae, termed 'homogonic' to distinguish them from the 'heterogonic' free-living, sexual generation, may become infective or may moult into free-living males and females. This, inevitably, strongly fosters the capacity to cause infection, especially as the free-living forms can produce further infective types. Infective larvae

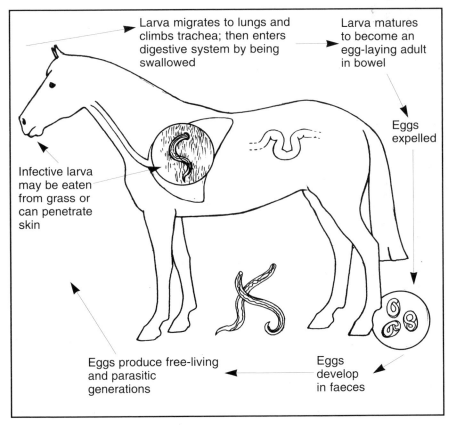

Larva migrates to lungs and climbs trachea; then enters digestive system by being swallowed

Larva matures to become an egg-laying adult in bowel

Eggs expelled

Infective larva may be eaten from grass or can penetrate skin

Eggs produce free-living and parasitic generations

Eggs develop in faeces

*Life cycle of threadworm*

may enter the host by penetrating the skin or the mucous membrane of the mouth.

A more significant line is the transmission of migrating larvae from mare to foal through the milk. There is some suggestion that this may be implicated in foaling-heat scours; though this is not established, it could be a contributory factor at times; but the pattern of foaling-heat scours generally does not lend itself to this hypothesis.

## Identifying Features

Threadworms are filariform (hair-like) worms some 8mm to 10mm long. They are identified by their anatomical details, especially the shape and length of the oesophagus.

## Clinical Signs

Infection with *S. westeri* involves migration to the lungs after entering the host, from which larvae travel up the trachea and are swallowed. This phase of infection may result in respiratory distress and inevitably involves a degree of haemorrhage in the process. The worms mature in the small intestine.

There is also the possibility of skin irritation caused by penetration. Severe damage to the lining of the small intestine may occur in heavy infestations, with consequent digestive disruption. Immunity occurs at an early stage in some individuals, though young animals diseased with heavy burdens are emaciated and diarrhoeic. Adult horses may have heavy burdens without any evident clinical sign.

The prepatent period of infection is only five to seven days and migrat-

*Adult threadworm*

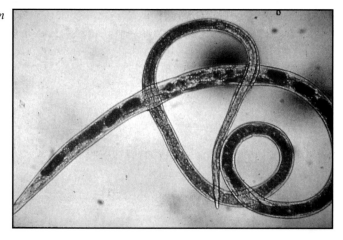

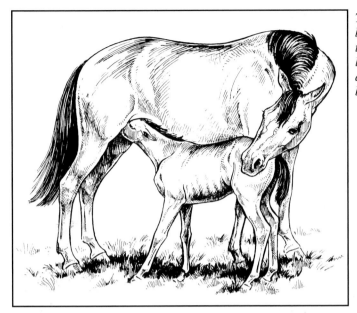

*The foal may be infected with threadworm larvae in milk as soon as it is born*

ing larvae can cross through to the mammary gland to infect suckling foals via the milk, a most important feature of this disease.

S. *westeri* is world-wide in distribution and development of infective larvae is greatly favoured by climatic conditions.

**Diagnosis**
Diagnosis is based on the presence of eggs and larvae in the faeces.

**Control**
Control of free-living generations is vital and best achieved by removing droppings and regular resting of pastures. Pre-foaling (or foaling day) worming of mares is vital to prevent infection of foals from the milk. Foals may shed eggs as early as two weeks of age and may develop diarrhoea at the time, which may coincide with the foaling-heat. Heavy infections of foals last for as long as ten weeks and lighter infections may persist even longer.

**Treatment**
S. *westeri* is susceptible to ivermectin, also to cambendazole. Oxibendazole has been found effective at 1.5 times the normal dosage. Fenbendazole at increased dosage rates is used (refer to manufacturer's literature). Febental, available in the USA, is used at increased dosage rates.

- The presence of free-living and parasitic generations may increase pasture larva counts
- *Strongyloides* is unique in being transferred from mare to foal in milk
- Prepatent period is five to seven days
- Foals may pass eggs in their faeces as early as ten days
- Development of infective larvae is greatly helped by warm, humid conditions
- Pasture hygiene is an important aspect of control

*Summary chart: threadworm*

# Lungworm (*Dictyocaulus*)

*Dictyocaulus arnfieldi* are elongated roundworms that can measure as long as 7cm in the donkey (considered the natural host). In horses, most developing larvae fail to reach sexual maturity and egg-laying – though the clinical effect is much more noticeable than in the donkey, which may fail to show external signs even with heavy burdens. Donkeys are said to be 'reservoir hosts' for horses with regard to this parasite.

Migrating larvae in the horse often provoke severe tissue reactions. *D. arnfieldi* is world-wide in distribution and is favoured in its development by heavy rainfall.

### Life Cycle

There is a typical, direct nematode life cycle. Eggs are laid by mature worms in the bronchi, from which they are carried (or coughed) up the trachea to the oesophagus. Here they are swallowed and passed out in the faeces.

The prepatent period for the infection is about five to six weeks. Ingested infective larvae penetrate the bowel and migrate to the lungs via the lymphatics and blood circulation, where they mature to the adult stage. The predeliction site is the bronchi and bronchioles of the lungs.

### Identifying Features

The male of the species has a well developed, though small, bursa. The buccal capsule is small.

### Clinical Signs

Coughing is a feature of the condition in horses though it has been established that donkeys with even heavy burdens may show no sign of infection. The pathological effect of parasites breaking into the lungs and residing in the bronchial lumen is mucus production, breathing difficulties, coughing and inappetence. There may be an accompanying pneumonia and heavy infestations are capable of causing death, especially in foals. The predominant clinical sign in the horse is chronic coughing. Severe disease may be complicated by the presence of other parasites in the bowel.

### Diagnosis

Diagnosis may be hindered by the absence of recognisable eggs or larvae in the faeces, and a presumptive diagnosis only reached on the basis of response to worm therapy.

Eggs are embryonated when laid. They hatch almost immediately, so only larvae are found on faecal examination.

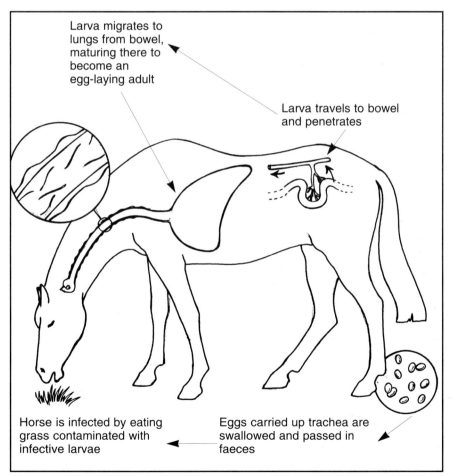

Larva migrates to lungs from bowel, maturing there to become an egg-laying adult

Larva travels to bowel and penetrates

Horse is infected by eating grass contaminated with infective larvae

Eggs carried up trachea are swallowed and passed in faeces

*Life cycle of lungworm*

Diagnosis can be aided by endoscopy. Tracheal washings can produce large numbers of eggs or larvae in patent infections.

### Control
Control requires strict supervision of horse/donkey contact so as to avoid inadvertant build up. Also, adult horses may harbour mild, non-clinical burdens which manage to develop to maturity and thus endanger younger animals. Lungworm larvae are sensitive to drying and direct sunlight, so that infected pastures will be safer if well drained. Where rain encourages larval build up, horses should be moved to fresh ground. Frequent removal of faeces from pasture is also a help. Regular dosing is required.

*D. arnfieldi* larvae utilise the fungus *Pilobolus* to reach vegetation from the faeces. The fungus develops like a balloon with an internal build-up of liquid and it tends to rupture in the middle of the day. The larvae are in this way thrown up to some 3m from the faecal pad where they find their way onto blades of grass.

It should be appreciated that lungworm is not the problem in horses that it can be in cattle. The often impaired life cycle influences pasture contamination and this parasite is not a major player in the routine annual cycle of events. Nevertheless, lungworm is a significant cause of disease where it does occur in horses and has to be taken into account in any situation where there is chronic coughing.

### Treatment
Ivermectin is effective against both mature and immature lungworms. Fenbendazole is recommended for use against adult stages of the worm; and levamisole is effective against the bovine lungworm but does not receive manufacturer's recommendations for use in horses. Levamisole is sometimes used in aqueous solution combined with piperazine against large strongyles, ascarids and pinworms.

---

- The donkey is often a symptomless carrier
- Adult horses may carry light infections without coughing
- Prepatent period is five to six weeks
- Infectious larvae develop in about five days

---

*Summary chart: lungworm*

# Horse Roundworm (*Parascaris*)

While all nematodes are roundworms, *Parascaris equorum* is allowed the common title of horse roundworm. It is probably the most striking roundworm seen on post-mortem examination, because of its large, fleshy size, the strength of its integument and its shining white colour. Adult *Parascaris* can measure as much as 50cm in length.

## Life Cycle

*Parascaris* has a direct life cycle. Second-stage larvae develop to infectivity on pasture within the egg in from ten days to six weeks. These eggs, which are ingested by the host, are notably durable, can resist adverse weather conditions and may over-winter on pasture.

Larvae hatch within the host and penetrate the wall of the small intestine from whence they migrate via the circulatory system to the liver and

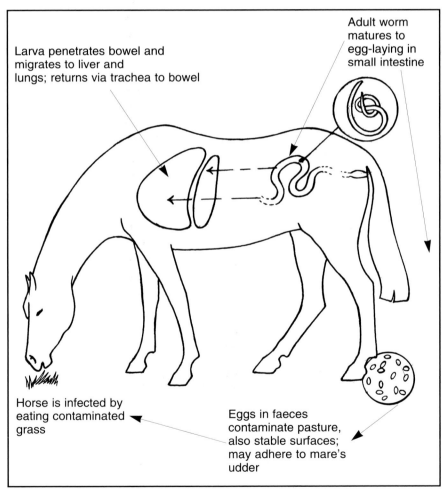

Larva penetrates bowel and migrates to liver and lungs; returns via trachea to bowel

Adult worm matures to egg-laying in small intestine

Horse is infected by eating contaminated grass

Eggs in faeces contaminate pasture, also stable surfaces; may adhere to mare's udder

*Life cycle of horse roundworm*

*The resistant eggs of horse roundworm*

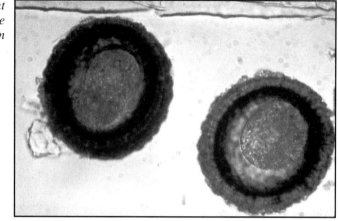

lungs. (They reach the liver in about two days and the lungs about one week later). After moulting in the lungs, they break through to the air passages and travel up the trachea. From here they find their way to the small intestine where they complete a final moult and mature to egg-laying adults. They reach the intestine in about four weeks after infection and at that stage are only 2mm long. Adult males measure about 25cm, females 50cm.

The prepatent period is about 11 weeks.

Eggs are found in the faeces of foals as young as 80 days, meaning that infection may occur soon after birth. There is no evidence of transmission from the dam, although eggs may adhere to the exterior of the mammary gland and be ingested by the foal from there.

The level of infection is influenced by the fecundity of the female and the resistance of the egg. Females may lay as many as 200,000 eggs per day, which are covered by a thick sticky layer that adheres to many surfaces and are viable for years. Embryonation takes weeks or months, depending on temperature. Eggs may adhere to indoor surfaces and are almost impossible to eliminate fully.

*Parascaris* worms are world-wide in distribution.

**Identifying Features**
Size and colour are the predominant gross characteristics. There is a prominent head with three lips.

**Clinical Signs**
There are two clinical expressions of *Parascaris* disease in the foal – the

respiratory form (occurs at between three and four weeks after infection) and the intestinal form (occurs later).

This worm is especially significant in the young foal, where symptoms may include weight loss, poor coat and swollen abdomen. Clumps of adult worms may gather to virtually block the small intestine or bile duct. Gut perforation sometimes occurs. Foals kept under intensive conditions are at greatest risk and may develop very large burdens. Haemorrhage in the lungs may be caused by the appearance there of large numbers of migrating worms.

There is also the effect of allergic type reactions after the host has become sensitised to the worm. These may only take a matter of weeks to develop after the intial infection and can greatly add to the severity of the clinical symptoms.

The presence of large numbers of worms in the intestine may cause acute enteritis (as seen post-mortem) and diarrhoea or constipation may ensue as a clinical expression of this. There may be coughing, fever, and pneumonia as a consequence of lung migration. The simultaneous migration of large numbers of larvae up the air passages may give rise to a nasal discharge.

Mature horses are generally resistant and this resistance starts to express itself after about six months of age.

**Diagnosis**
Diagnosis is suspected in the case of foals showing typical signs. It is confirmed by the presence of eggs in the faeces.

**Control**
The main purpose of control is to prevent or limit infection in foals. Pregnant mares should be treated with suitable drugs so as to counter this infection and then be moved to clean pastures for foaling. Frequent removal of manure from pastures is an essential part of management. Larva containing eggs will die in the fermenting conditions that develop in muck-heaps, but eggs on pasture are very resistant to drying out.

It is also advised to bathe the udder and teats of pre-foaling mares to remove eggs (which may be acquired by lying on polluted soils). Thorough disinfection of the foaling box is also sensible (although eggs are resistant to chemicals and are best removed, using high pressure or steam cleaning, from walls, doors and fittings).

The most difficult factors in control of this disease are the continued low-level infection of horses of all ages and the special resistance of *Parascaris* eggs. The condition is not helped either by the common tendency for foals to eat their mother's droppings or by the propensity of eggs to adhere to walls, mangers and buckets.

**Treatment**
Fenbendazole, ivermectin and pyrantel are all effective against the adult stages of this worm. Most of the other benzimidazole drugs are also effective as is piperazine either alone or in conjunction with thiabendazole or levamisole.

---

- *Parascaris* is the most significant parasite of foals up to six months
- Eggs are very resistant and may survive for years
- Foals may ingest eggs from mares' udders and stable surfaces
- Eggs become infective in a period between ten days and six weeks
- Prepatent period is about eleven weeks
- Well-composted manure kills eggs
- Female worms lay large numbers of eggs

---

*Summary chart: horse roundworm*

# Hairworm (*Trichostrongylus*)

*Trichostrongylus axei* is a small worm about 0.5cm in length. Its predeliction site is the horse's stomach glands and small intestine. It contributes to mixed worm infections and is a significant parasite of cattle and sheep, thus warranting major consideration in deciding on mixed grazing regimens.

The parasite is found in most countries of temperate climate and has added significance in that infective larvae are able to overwinter on pasture.

**Life Cycle**
There is a typical direct nematode life cycle. First-stage larvae hatch in one to two days; they and second-stage larvae live on microorganisms in faeces. Third-stage larvae are infective, a stage that develops on pasture in about four to six days after emergence from the host. This depends on climatic conditions, larvae emerging from the faeces and finding their way to the soil and vegetation. The prepatent period is three weeks.

**Identifying Features**
Males have a bursa and there is almost no buccal capsule. Females do not

lay large numbers of eggs, but this is offset by the nature of the worm and the fact that it parasitises cattle and sheep as well as horses.

**Clinical Signs**

The presence of *T. axei* irritates the lining of the stomach, causing plaque formation, sometimes erosion and blood loss. Chronic diarrhoea may be a consequence of functional damage to the gut wall and anaemia results from blood loss. Plasma proteins leak into the lumen of the stomach further complicating the picture. Affected animals lose weight and can develop dependent oedema.

**Diagnosis**

Positive identification is dependent on larval culture, so diagnosis is not possible on the basis of eggs in faeces alone.

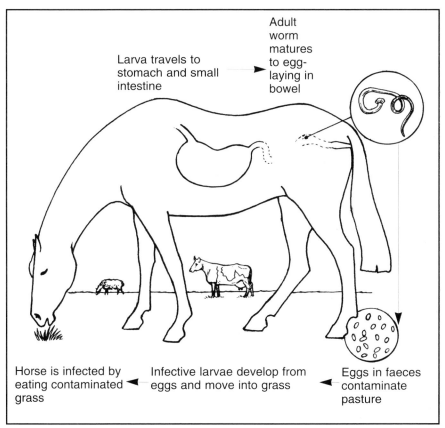

*Life cycle of hairworm. Mixed grazing may increase infection*

*Adult hairworm*

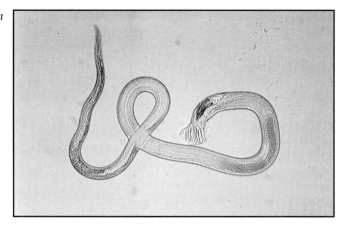

*Hairworm lesions from the stomach of a donkey*

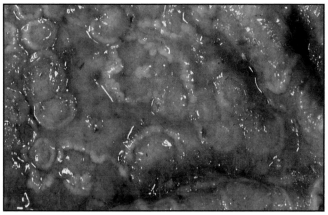

However, the diagnosis in foals, particularly, will be suggested by the nature of the faeces (diarrhoea), and a history of intensive grazing on pasture that also supports cattle and/or sheep.

## Control

Foals are very susceptible to *T. axei* infection and repeated treatment is necessary. Mares should be treated before foaling and moved to clean pastures where they can avoid both overcrowding and those pastures which are intensively grazed by cattle and sheep. Removal of faeces from mare and foal paddocks is necessary and it is sometimes wise to plough grazing areas with dense ground cover that encourage the over-wintering of larvae.

*T. axei* infective larvae can overwinter because they are highly resistant to cold. The surviving generation will get killed off with strong sunshine, but not before infecting a new generation of hosts, thus contributing to a build-up of worms during the summer and the development of another population of overwintering larvae. The management of grazing is very important, especially where there are cattle and sheep. However, there is a possiblity that special strains only infect given hosts and *T. axei* is not a cause of major disease in adult horses under normal conditions. Still, heavy burdens can occur and it is important to eliminate any secondary factors – for example, lowered resistance which may ensue from environmental factors, nutrition or poor management practices.

**Treatment**

Ivermectin is effective against the adult stage of *T. axei*. Febental, at increased dosage rates, shows some effect and benzimidazole wormers have proven efficacy against the worm in cattle.

---

- *Trichostrongylus* is also a parasite of cattle and sheep
- Larvae are durable and can over-winter
- *Trichostrongylus* is an important disease of foals
- Breaking ground cover by harrowing, topping or ploughing helps to expose larvae to destruction
- Prepatent period is three weeks
- Infective larvae develop in four to six days

---

*Summary chart: hairworm*

# Pinworm (*Oxyuris*)

The male of the pinworm, *Oxyuris equi*, measures only 10mm to 12mm in length while the female, which has a long, pin-like tail, is much larger and may be 10cm or longer. Pinworm larvae are plug feeders, thus causing considerable damage to the bowel. Adult worms feed only on intestinal contents.

Pinworms have a world-wide distribution.

**Life Cycle**

The female migrates from the horse's large intestine to the anus and lays her eggs on the skin of the perineum around it. Eggs are laid in sticky clumps and each of these may contain as many as 50,000 eggs which, covered in a viscous, sticky fluid, become infective in three to five days,

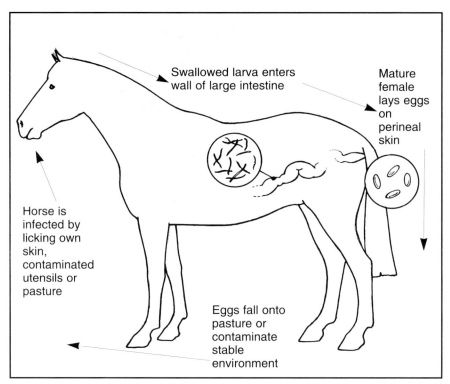

*Life cycle of pinworm*

depending on external temperatures. They detach in flakes of the dried fluid to contaminate the stable or ground. They may also drop into feed or water containers, or animals may be directly infected by biting at the local tissue irritation caused by the fluid.

Ingested larvae penetrate the wall of the large intestine where they reach maturity in four to five months.

### Identifying Features
The long tail of the female is characteristic, and there is a large buccal capsule.

### Clinical Signs
Loss of condition occurs in heavy infestations, due as much to scratching and local irritation as to intestinal damage, which may extend to ulceration. Infected horses scratch consistently, fail to thrive and may bear self-inflicted wounds. The effect on the tail may cause hair loss, but it is

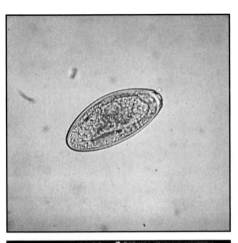

*Pinworm egg*

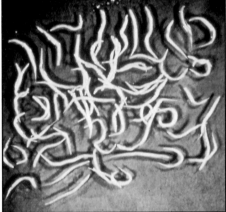

*Adult pinworms*

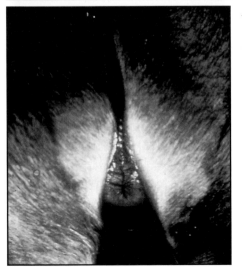

*Pinworm eggs under the horse's tail*

important not to confuse the symptoms with sweet-itch, also selenium toxicity; tail rubbing can also sometimes amount to little more than a stable habit. In severe cases there may be anorexia and anxiety.

## Diagnosis

The sight of pale yellow egg-containing fluid about the perineum is diagnostic of this infection. The eggs can be collected by using a transparent adhesive tape and identified under a microscope in a laboratory. Scratching is not an essential sign as horses may have the infection without any trace of tail irritation.

## Control

Hygiene is important, especially within the stable. Cleanliness of buckets and other containers must be ensured, and occasional steam-cleaning, especially of recesses and porous surfaces, is important. Infection is also possible through eating contaminated feed and bedding.

Inevitably, also, good grooming is an essential feature of control and involves the recognition of the offensive material on the perineum and its removal.

## Treatment

Adult worms are susceptible to most modern anthelmintics including pyrantel, ivermectin and fenbendazole.

---

- Clumps of eggs are seen on perinaeum in sticky yellow mucus that dries and falls off in flakes
- Tail irritation is also a feature of conditions like sweet-itch
- Prepatent period is four to five months
- Eggs are infective in three to five days
- Stable hygiene is important with this parasite
- While females lay large numbers of eggs this worm is not a major disease agent in horses

---

*Summary chart: pinworm*

# Neck Threadworm (*Onchocerca*)

*Onchocerca cervicalis* worms are long and coiled, males being between 5cm and 6cm and females growing up to 30cm in length. Microfilariae (the embryonic form of larva in this species) are about 0.25mm long. The very slender, thread-like worm, *O. cervicalis*, is difficult to identify in tissues because of its filamentous nature.

## Life Cycle

*O. cervicalis* has an indirect life cycle, the intermediate host being a biting fly, *Culicoides nubeculosus*, which feeds on the horse's abdominal midline.

The adult female worm is found in the ligamentum nuchae, the extensive ligament that supports the head from the withers of the horse. She does not lay eggs but gives birth to mobile embryos, microfilariae. These are found in subcutaneous lymph tissues, mainly on the underside of the horse's body, face (including the conjunctiva), and inside of the limbs, where they are ingested by feeding flies. Infective larvae develop within these insects and are present in their mouthparts 24 days later, so gaining entry to new hosts as the flies feed again. The prepatent period is one month.

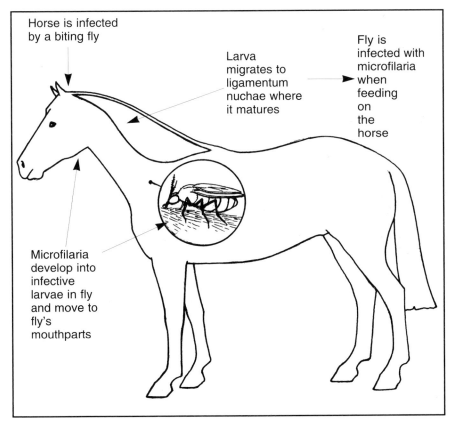

*Life cycle of neck threadworm*

*Neck threadworm microfilariae in tissues* (arrowed)

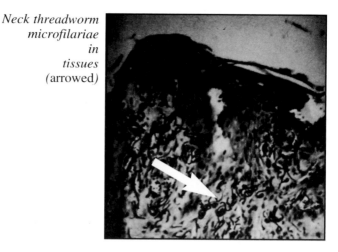

O. *reticulata* is found in the tendons and ligaments of the horse's lower forelimb particularly.

The worm is distributed world-wide. However, its clinical significance in both the UK and Ireland is unclear.

**Identifying Features**

The length and filamentous nature of the adult females is characteristic. Also, the production of microfilariae, as opposed to eggs, has special significance. Identification of microfilariae, which may be found in skin biopsies, is a matter for laboratory specialists.

**Clinical Signs**

Heavy burdens are debilitating and can influence movement of the part they parasitise. Adult worms in ligaments and tendons may cause swelling and pain. Nodules may develop where worms have died and the tissues calcify. Microfilariae may infiltrate the eye and cause irritation, and even blindness. Lameness may result from their effect on leg tendons and ligaments.

Local skin irritation is caused by the presence of microfilariae, but it also results from allergic reactions to their presence. Skin lesions are found on the horse's face, neck, shoulders and breast and can be intensely itchy.

**Diagnosis**

Microfilariae may be found in skin samples taken and soaked in saline for a number of hours. However, it is possible for horses to be infected with this parasite without showing clinical signs. Identificiation of microfilariae in some cases will therefore not necessarily explain existing skin lesions.

### Control

Where it is practical, control of the insect intermediate host is worthy of consideration. However, the effect of some modern anthelmintics against the microfilariae means that judicious treatment, especially related to the timing of the fly season, might help to greatly reduce the problems caused by *O. cervicalis*.

### Treatment

Adult *Onchocerca* may persist in the ligamentum nuchae for the life of the horse and no drug to date is effective in eliminating them fully. Microfilariae are susceptible to some modern anthelmintics, for example, ivermectin, levamisole and diethylcarbamazine. It must be considered, however that destruction of microfilariae in local tissues may result in adverse host reactions, and this could be particularly significant in relation to the eye.

---

- Predilection site for adult worm is the ligamentum nuchae (also other ligaments and tendons)
- Intermediate host is a biting fly
- Females produce microfilariae rather than eggs
- Prepatent period is one month
- Larvae are infective within fly in three weeks
- *Onchocerca* is not considered a major cause of disease

---

*Summary chart: neck threadworm*

# Abdominal Worm (*Setaria*)

*Setaria equina* is a long slender worm, with males measuring about 8cm and females up to 13cm. It has an indirect life cycle, like *Onchocerca*, the intermediate host being a mosquito, and also produces microfilariae which are 0.25mm long.

This parasite is common in warmer areas of the world, and seldom seen in moderate climates where the intermediate host does not live.

### Life Cycle

Larvae are produced by adult worms in body cavities from whence they

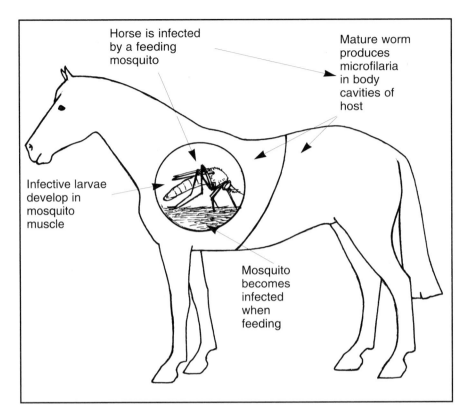

*Life cycle of abdominal worm*

circulate in the blood and are taken up by mosquitoes, including those of *Aedes* and *Culex* species, when feeding. Infective larvae develop in mosquito muscle in about two weeks and are transferred to horses when infected mosquitoes feed again. The prepatent period is eight to ten-months.

## Identifying Features
Adult worms are more slender than *Parascaris* and do not have the same type of mouth. The tail of the male is corkscrew shaped, this being a characteristic of filarial worms. Adult *Setaria* have small mouths.

## Clinical Signs
Adult worms are parasites of serous membranes and live in the cavity of the abdomen, but are occasionally found in the lungs, liver, scrotum and

eyes. In the abdomen, they are thought to cause little trouble, but worms in the eye may have a serious effect on sight even leading to blindness. They may also find their way to the brain and spinal cord, especially *Setaria* species of sheep or cattle that find their way into a horse, where they can cause a type of encephalomyelitis seen in the Far East.

**Diagnosis**
Diagnosis depends on finding microfilariae in the blood or adult worms on post-mortem examination.

**Control**
Control is helped by the control of mosquitoes.

**Treatment**
Adult worms in the abdomen generally cause little or no symptoms, except where large burdens are carried, but there are few records of any success in treating these. Eye problems caused by *Setaria* can lead to blindness and may have to be dealt with surgically for any hope of success.

---

- *Setaria* occurs in countries where mosquitoes exist
- Fly control is important where *Setaria* occurs
- Prepatent period is eight to ten months
- Infective larvae develop within mosquito in two weeks
- Aberrant larvae may cause eye lesions or symptoms related to the central nervous system

---

*Summary chart: abdominal worm*

# Eyeworm (*Thelazia*)

Adult eyeworms parasitise the tear ducts of the horse's upper and third eyelids and conjunctival sac. *Thelazia lacrymalis* may reach as long as 1.5cm in the adult stage.

Surveys have shown that as many as 30 per cent of horses in the UK are infected.

**Life Cycle**
The female lays eggs containing larvae into the tears and these are picked up by a fly intermediate host (for example, *Musca autumnalis*) and are

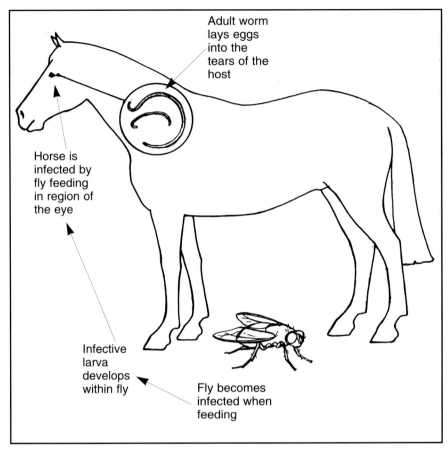

*Life-cycle of eyeworm*

infective within that host after 30 days. The eggs are thus transferred to the eyes of other horses when the fly feeds again.

**Identifying Features**
*Thelazia* is a long, slender worm whose predilection site is the eye.

**Clinical Signs**
Small numbers of worms may produce little damage, but heavy infesta-

tions cause severe irritation and local tissue damage and can sometimes lead to blindness. Secondary bacterial infection is also not unusual.

## Diagnosis
Diagnosis depends on recognition of the adult worm, or of the larvae in tears.

## Control
Fly control depends on the use of insecticides, of good hygiene, and of methods like screening to protect horses from fly worry.

## Treatment
Adult worms may be removed under local anaesthesia by qualified veterinary personnel. Treatment in cattle is tetramisole by subcutaneous injection, or levamisole, which can also be used as a 1 per cent solution

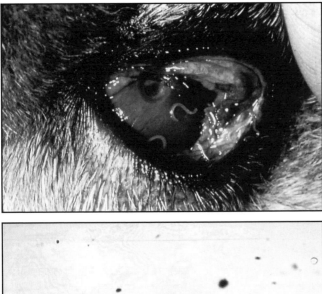

*Adult eyeworm in the eye*

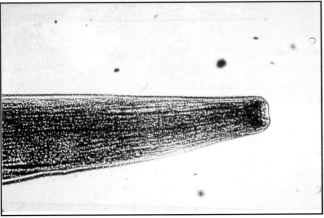

*Anterior end of eyeworm adult*

into the eye. (Do *not* attempt any such procedure; consult your vet if the condition is suspected.)

---

- In the UK, 30 per cent of horses are said to be affected with *Thelazia*, but clinical eye disease is not seen in most cases
- Most common in fly season
- Infective larvae develop within fly in 30 days

---

*Summary chart: eyeworm*

# Stomach Worms (*Habronema and Draschia*)

The worms, *Habronema muscae, Habronema microstoma* and *Draschia megastoma,* are all stomach worms. The adults are whitish in colour and measure from 1cm to 3.5cm in length. Females lay small numbers of eggs. They are particularly significant as the cause of 'summer sores', or cutaneous habronemiasis. A seasonal occurrence is directly related to the life of the fly vectors.

## Life Cycle
Eggs are laid from which larvae emerge quickly and these are ingested by housefly or stable fly maggots that develop in manure. These larvae become infective within the maggot in about one week, about the same time as the adult fly emerges from its pupa. The larvae migrate to the fly's head, from whence they are deposited on moist areas like the lips, nostrils and prepuce, also about wounds on horses as the flies feed. Once licked and swallowed by the host the larvae develop to maturity in the stomach. When the larvae are deposited on wounds or broken skin the life cycle is arrested and summer sores, which mainly occur in warm climates, develop.

## Identifying Features
Male worms bear a flat spiral tail. The head is distinct and has lips and a tooth. *Habronema* species are larger than *Draschia.*

## Clinical Signs
Surface lesions are marked by a rapid production of granulation tissue that refuses to resolve during the fly season. Itching is intense and may

lead to self-inflicted further injury. The extent of this may relate to hyper-sensitivity to the larvae.

Larvae infecting wounds may migrate and feed, extending the size of the wound and delaying healing. These larvae do not complete their life cycle. Such infections may heal in winter but recur when flies are again prevalent. Larvae deposited in the eye cause wart-like lesions, with watering eyes. Ulcerated nodules may appear near the medial canthus of the eye.

Lesions also occur at the urethral process, prepuce, ventral body and legs. Areas which are moist attract flies and are prone to infection.

Infection of the digestive system can also occur by ingestion of flies with water or feed. The adult worms reside on the lining of the stomach under thick plugs of mucus and may be diagnosed on faecal examination

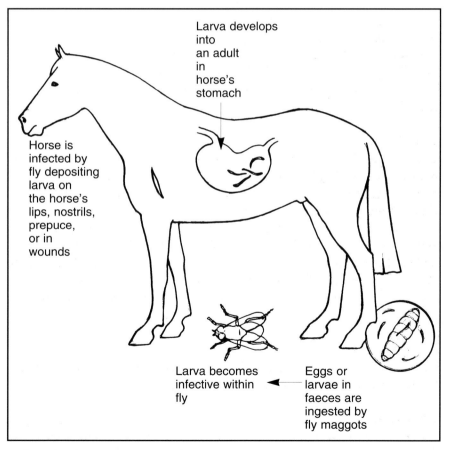

*Life cycle of stomach worm*

through the presence of eggs, larvae and the like. They do not cause great harm but larvae in the eye or associated with wounds may cause severe irritation.

*D. megastoma* causes the formation of nodules in the horse's stomach which develop into tumour-like growths, and these may rupture or can block the passage of food from the stomach into the small intestine. Adult worms may affect digestion if present in large numbers.

### Diagnosis

Where chronic granulomatous development occurs in wounds which are refractory to treatment, skin scrapings may expose the presence of larvae. Lesions close to the eye are not unusual and their character and persistence suggest the nature of the condition.

Eggs or larvae may be found in the faeces.

### Control

The only method of control is the elimination of adult worms through anthelmintic treatment as well as effective fly control where this is possible. Wounds should be treated with fly-repellants.

### Treatment

The use of ivermectin orally may well kill the larvae in local wounds. It has proven efficacy against adult worms in the stomach. Further treatment would include normal wound hygiene, the control of granulation tissue and the prevention of further larval contamination by fly control. Lesions in the region of the eye might require surgery in order to prevent more serious complications.

---

- *Habronema* only occurs in warmer climates
- Adult worms may cause tumour-like growths in stomach but are susceptible to treatment
- Skin lesions caused by larvae are difficult to treat
- Infective larvae develop within fly in one week

---

*Summary chart: stomach worms*

## Gullet Worm (*Gonglyonema*)

A parasite of the horse's oesophagus, *Gonglyonema pulchrum* reaches as much as 14.5cm in length and is identified by the presence of rows of wart-like thickenings, especially at its upper end.

Distribution is said to be world-wide, but the parasite has little known clinical significance other than a degree of mild oesophageal irritation.

**Life Cycle**
Eggs passed in faeces are ingested by dung beetles in which they hatch and develop to the infective stage in about one month. Horses are infected by eating the beetles, but the route of migration to the oesophagus is not understood.

The mature worm becomes embedded in the lining of the oesophagus.

**Identifying Features**
Gongylonema is a particularly long worm that possesses rows of nodu-

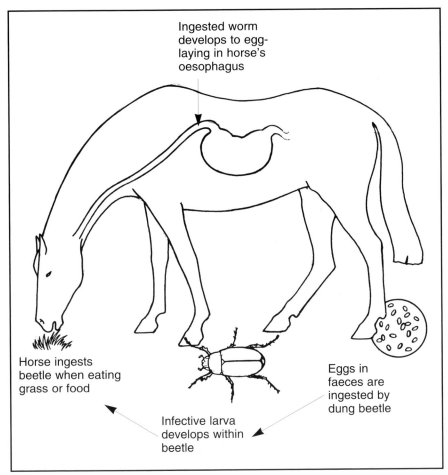

*Life-cycle of gullet worm*

lar thickenings on its upper end. Its predeliction site is the host's oesophagus.

**Diagnosis**
Diagnosis depends on finding eggs in the faeces or adult worms in the oesophagus on post-mortem examination.

**Control**
The best form of control is removal of dung from the grazing areas of horses.

**Treatment**
Little is recorded about treatment for this parasite.

---

- Infective larvae develop within beetle in about one month
- This parasite is considered virtually harmless

---

*Summary chart: gullet worm*

We now turn to the four biological groupings identified earlier: *Cestoda*, *Trematoda*, *Protozoa*, and *Insecta*. The clinical effects of the parasites within the first three groups are less significant than those caused by roundworms. However, tapeworms and fluke are themselves recognised causes of disease in horses, sometimes of serious consequence, while the influence of protozoan disease is not great in temperate climates.

# Cestodes

The only cestodes significant to the horse are the tapeworms, *Anoplocephala perfoliata* and *Anoplocephala magna*. The adult parasite can develop to as long as 80cm in the case of *A. magna* and is about 2cm wide. The anterior end (called the scolex) is spherical, unarmed, and has four suckers. The body of the worm consists of segments (proglottids) which are broad and thin and these develop from behind the scolex. Segments of *A. perfoliata* are very short and closely attached to each other.

**Tapeworms**

Equine tapeworms are found on a world-wide basis and recent reports from both the UK and the USA suggest that in excess of 50 per cent of horses may be affected. Some opinion holds that this has only happened since the introduction of ivermectin to the market. The suggestion is that the effectiveness of this drug has eliminated other worms to the extent that tapeworms, which are not killed by the drug, are given advantage; however, modern work carried out in Louisiana State University refutes this theory.

## Life Cycle

The proglottids at the distal end of the tapeworm become enlarged with eggs and are finally released and passed out in the faeces. These eggs are released as the proglottids decompose and are ingested by intermediate hosts. Larvae become infective within the intermediate host, the oribatid mite, within two to four months.

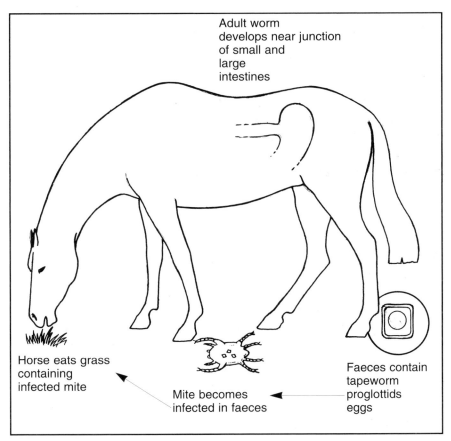

Life cycle of tapeworm

*Adult tapeworms showing the scolex at the narrow end; the cross-stripes mark the divisions of the proglottids*

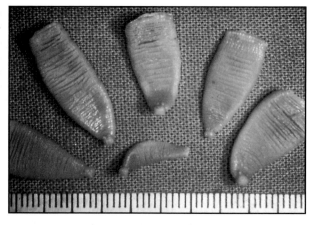

*Tapeworm eggs*

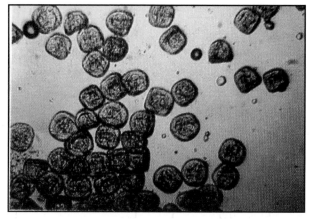

*The oribatid mite*

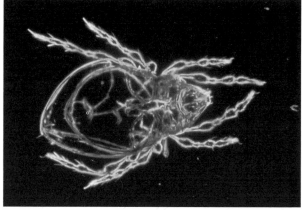

After these mites are eaten by grazing horses, larvae develop to maturity within the lower small intestine, the caecum and colon (*A. perfoliata*) of the host within four to six weeks. *A. magna* lives almost exclusively in the small intestine. *Paranoplocephala mamillana* occurs in the small intestine and stomach and is the smallest of these worms, reaching only about 3cm adult size.

**Identifying Features**
Tapeworms are recognised by their segmented nature and great length. The scolex contains four suckers.

**Clinical Signs**
While the tapeworm was not formerly considered to have a great clinical significance, this idea has changed in recent years and there is no doubt that large worm burdens develop which cannot be beneficial to the host. In animals in already poor condition they may act as a futher stress and their presence in mixed parasite infections is also likely to be harmful.

Tapeworms compete with the host for food and nutrients and this explains their effect when present in large numbers. They may also cause intestinal irritation, leading to thickening of the gut wall, ulcer formation and possible perforation. Other complications may follow and intestinal blockage may result from accumulations of tapeworms at the junction of the small intestine and caecum. Loss of weight, colic and persistent diarrhoea are symptoms which have been attributed to this disease.

**Diagnosis**
Diagnosis depends on the identification of eggs in the faeces, or tapeworm segments, or on the presence of adult worms in the bowel post-mortem. However, negative faecal results can occur where there are significant numbers of tapeworms in the bowel.

**Control**
Control involves the regular use of drugs to which the parasite is sensitive, coupled with good pasture hygiene.

**Treatment**
Pyrantel is effective at twice the normal dosage rate, and is recommended at this rate by manufacturers. Dichlorophene, available in the USA, is also effective against equine tapeworms. Mebendazole at increased dosage rates has shown some effect against *Anoplocephala* but findings were not consistent.

Treatment should be given at winter stabling and when horses are at grass for about three months.

---

- In excess of 50 per cent of horses may be infected
- Tapeworms are thought to be capable of causing serious disease
- Some opinion believes that this may result from faulty medication procedures
- Prepatent period is four to six weeks
- Infective larvae develop in mite in two to four months

---

*Summary chart: tapeworms*

## Other Tapeworms

The horse also acts as an intermediate host for *Echinococcus granulosus* and can harbour the metacestodes of *Taenia hydatigena* and *Taenia multiceps* (all of which are recognised parasites of ruminants). These structures develop as bladder-like cysts which may find their way to the brain or can develop in organs such as the liver. By the very size they develop to, pressure can be placed on neighbouring organs, thus interfering with their normal purpose; they are usually harmless in the lungs and liver.

# Trematodes

The most common trematode found in the horse is the liver fluke, *Fasciola hepatica*, a parasite of cattle and sheep. There is one intermediate host, a freshwater snail, *Limnaea truncatula*. The lancet fluke, *Dicrocoelium dendriticum* also occurs in parts of Europe, but differs in there being two intermediate hosts, a snail and a brown ant.

## Liver Fluke

Fluke are found world-wide in areas that provide a suitable habitat for the snail – the wetter parts of most temperate areas. A survey carried out in Ireland showed 77 per cent of horses and 91 per cent of donkeys to be affected. The comparative figures in the UK were 0.1 per cent (horses) and 33 per cent (donkeys) although the figure for horses might be conservative in some situations.

In hot climates, *F. gigantica* occurs, which may grow to 7.5cm in length. This parasite too may infest horses. *F. magna*, measuring up to 10cm x 3cm, is a deer parasite in North America and is also occasionally found in horses.

## Life Cycle

Adult fluke lay eggs in the liver and these are carried to the intestine in the bile. They hatch when passed in the faeces, and the immature fluke (called a miracidium at this stage) penetrate into a snail for the continuation of its life cycle.

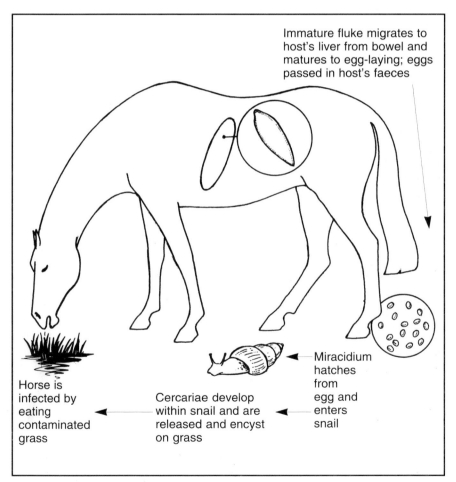

Immature fluke migrates to host's liver from bowel and matures to egg-laying; eggs passed in host's faeces

Horse is infected by eating contaminated grass

Cercariae develop within snail and are released and encyst on grass

Miracidium hatches from egg and enters snail

*Life cycle of liver fluke*

The egg must fall into water for the miracidium to develop. This process takes two to four weeks at summer temperatures. The miracidium then swims about in search of the specific species of snail it requires, and will die in 24 hours if it fails to achieve this. The miracidium is covered in hair-like processes called cilia and it actively bores its way into the snail intermediate host.

Within the snail the miracidium loses its hairy coat and forms a sporocyst. This eventually leads to the production of rediae which in turn lead to the production of cercariae. All of these are stages in the development of the fluke, but the significant factor from a control viewpoint is the requirement for a habitat suitable to the intermediate host. Without this, the cycle is not complete and the fluke cannot gain entry to a new host.

Multiplication within the snail leads to the production of as many as 600 cercariae; these encyst on grass where they are eaten by grazing animals, including horses. The young parasites penetrate the host's gut and pass to the liver via the peritoneal cavity. For the following six to seven weeks, while growing rapidly, young fluke (called a marita at this stage) eat their way through the liver substance, leaving behind a trail of destruction which repairs by the formation of scar tissue. Mature fluke begin to lay eggs some six to twelve weeks after infection.

Development of cercariae takes one to two months at summer temperatures. They leave the snail and swim about in water until they migrate above water level to encyst (they are now called metacercariae, which are very resistant to drying) and await ingestion by grazing animals – which are most commonly ruminant, but include horses.

The whole life cycle can take three or four months under favourable conditions. The need for a suitable snail environment means that infective areas may occur only in specific fields or parts of fields where water lodges. Inevitably periods of drought will alter this. Small streams, ponds and marshy areas are usually suspect sources. Moist hay might act as source of infection, even in animals kept remote from an infected area.

The snail involved, an essential part of this cycle, can only exist in wet areas, around the edges of pools of fresh water. Although adult fluke may parasitise a number of different hosts, the cercariae are very host specific and will only develop in that snail species, therefore in areas inhabited by the snail. Fluke are also favoured when mild winters allow eggs and juvenile stages to survive on the land. Their proliferation is favoured by wet summers. In the horse, mature fluke are found in the bile duct.

**Identifying Features**
Adult worms are of a greyish-brown colour with an elongated, vaguely

triangular shape. The base of the triangle is the front end which bears a cone-shaped projection and the body tapers from behind this point.

**Clinical Signs**
Young fluke migrating through the liver cause tissue damage and in food-producing animals are responsible for rejection of livers at slaughter. This damage interferes with normal liver function and can cause acute destruction of tissue depending on the level of infection.

One of the most important clinical signs in the horse is anaemia. This results from ingestion of blood by the adult fluke and may also be affected by tissue damage causing haemorrhage as young fluke migrate through the liver. The situation is further aggravated by tissue irritation in the bile duct caused by the presence of mature fluke.

The result of chronic infection is weight loss and anaemia and this may lead to oedema. Other symptoms sometimes related to fluke infestation are passive leg-filling which quite often disappears after treatment with a suitable flukacide. Digestive disturbances are also reported and can contribute to lethargy and loss of performance.

**Diagnosis**
*Fasciola* eggs are found in the faeces, though a negative finding does not mean an animal is fluke free. In many cases, it is only a response to anti-fluke drugs that suggests a presumptive diagnosis in retrospect.

Adult fluke may be found in the liver on post-mortem examination.

A suspicion of fluke must always exist where horses graze areas on which fluke infected sheep and cattle exist. The horse, not being a natural

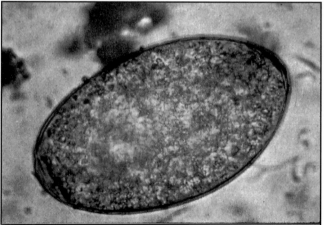

*Liver fluke egg*

host for this condition, may limit the life cycle of the fluke, and egg laying may be curtailed. Diagnosis in these situations is made more difficult. While the incidence may well be low, the condition does occur as a significant clinical problem in some horses. Inevitably, even the presence of moderate anaemia from fluke will affect performance, and the diagnosis is not always simply made, especially when no fluke eggs are found.

**Control**
Drainage of pastures to eliminate wet patches has a significant effect on this disease by preventing the proliferation of the specific snail intermediate host. It is also important to know that bought hay does not come from fluke infested land.

**Treatment**
Modern flukicide drugs are effective in treatment, the most common used in horses being oxyclozanide, used at a dose rate of not more than 100 ml for an adult animal. While the drug is not licensed for use in horses, the manufacturer does not see use as being a hazard in species other than cattle, sheep and pigs.

While it would be wrong to over-estimate the significance of this condition it would be equally wrong to dismiss its importance in clinical disease of the horse.

---

- Liver fluke should be considered when horses graze known infected pasture
- Intermediate host is a snail
- Drainage of land is an essential aspect of control
- Once diagnosed the condition can be treated
- Fluke disease is favoured by mild winters and wet summers
- The miracidium takes two to four weeks to develop
- Prepatent period is six to twelve weeks
- Cercariae take one to two months to develop

---

*Summary chart: liver fluke*

# Protozoan Infections

Coccidial infections (a type of protozoan disease) in horses are considered to be clinically rare. The nature of such diseases, as presently understood, suggests they are only likely to occur in immune-deficient foals and even then their ability to cause clinical disease appears limited. This may well understate the true situation.

It should be expected that the problem could arise on studfarms, or any other situation where horse populations are high and large numbers of foals are in daily contact.

*Coccidia* could quite easily become a complicating factor where hygiene is poor and viral and bacterial enteritis are already a problem. *Eimeria leuckarti*, a coccidial parasite, was found in 41 per cent of foals in a number of Kentucky studfarms. Oocysts first appeared in the faeces between 15 and 123 days and were shed for as long as four months. The condition is thought to be relatively harmless.

*E. leuckarti* reproduce in the lining cells of the intestine. This inevitably leads to a degree of cellular damage resulting in gross clinical signs – such as diarrhoea.

Oocysts are passed in the faeces and are approximately the same size as strongyle eggs. New hosts are infected by ingesting these oocysts after they have undergone a process called sporulation, which takes about two days. It must be understood that the presence of oocysts in faeces does not inevitably mean disease, although, in other species, infection can be severe even before oocysts have appeared.

The disease in horses is at present considered to be mild and of little significance. But it would be wise to consider that the potential for disease exists in intensive situations or where foals particularly are immune deficient.

## Other Protozoan Infections

There is a number of other protozoan infections which cause disease in horses. Some of the more important are discussed below.

### Babesia

A parasite of the red blood cells of horses, seen in the USA, *Babesia caballi* infection is also known as piroplasmosis. It is transmitted by the horse tick, *Dermacentor*.

### Klosiella

A parasite of the kidney of the horse, *Klosiella equi* is only likely to cause disease in immune deficient animals. It is also a coccidial organism similar to *Eimeria*.

## Equine Protozoan Myeloencephalitis

This disease occurs in the USA, but a great deal about its pathology is not understood. It is believed to be caused by the protozoan parasite, *Sarcocystis*.

## Dourine (*Trypanosoma*)

A protozoan parasite, *Trypanosoma equiperdum*, causes dourine in horses, a condition now rarely reported in North America. It occurs in Africa, Asia, parts of Europe, and Central and South America. The organism occurs in blood plasma, is elongated and tapers at both ends, measuring from 25–30 microns long by 1–2 microns wide.

The condition is primarily a venereal disease of horses, causing swelling and eruptions on the genital regions, from which pigment may disappear. There is usually a mucoid discharge. Plaque formation may also occur and be seen on the horse's neck and trunk.

A chronic form of the disease is associated with paresis, emaciation, fever and death.

Diagnosis is made on the basis of identification of the offending organisms in the blood. Infected horses are usually destroyed.

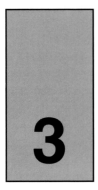

# 3 Pasture Management and Worm Control

Modern evidence has shown a growing resistance of some worms to particular anthelmintic drugs (especially the benzimidazole group) due to constant, routine use which may or may not be helped by lowering standards of pasture management relevant to worm exposure. The established procedure of routine dosing has relied too heavily on drug efficiency and has ignored the fact that increasing or uncontrolled pasture contamination might prove harmful in the long term.

Drug resistance is a consequence of intensification that accompanies a general increase in the horse population. The elementary belief was held that more efficient drugs might eliminate parasites completely, but this is not proving to be true and for very understandable reasons. Intelligent drug use should always keep in mind degree of exposure. In other words, if we allow a build-up of infective material on grazing lands, treated horses immediately re-infect after treatment (unless moved to fresh pasture) – there being no residual effect from the drugs we use. Therefore, horses may become subject to large intakes of worms on systems of even monthly or bi-monthly dosing. Added to this, drug resistance rules out any dream of worm eradication.

## Cyathostomes

Cyathostomes are thought to be one of the most significant modern worm groups of horses and it is with these that drug resistance (again, mainly with benzimidazole drugs) is particularly concerned. Cyathostomes are capable of building up huge burdens in grazing animals and the problem is exacerbated by improper drug use or poor pasture management. With

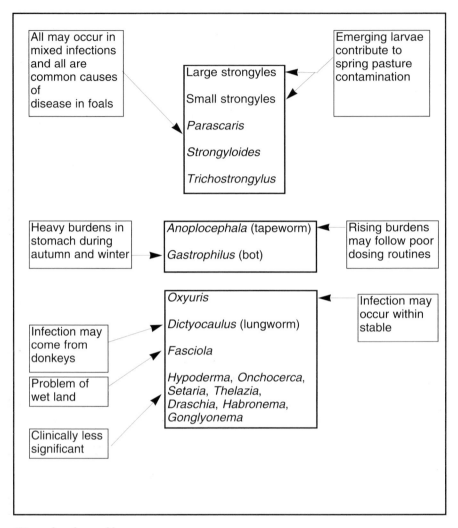

*Worm burdens of horses*

this infection there is a need to consider specific aspects of the parasite's life cycle as well as to use drugs which are effective within that context.

Colic is caused by cyathostomes as well as large strongyles and horses are known to die from the effects of this worm under particularly heavy infestations. As it happens, no single-dose anthelmintic has proven effective against encysted cyathostomes (although ivermectin reduces the incidence) and it is only after they have emerged from the bowel wall and caused their greatest harm that anthelmintics take effect. However, man-

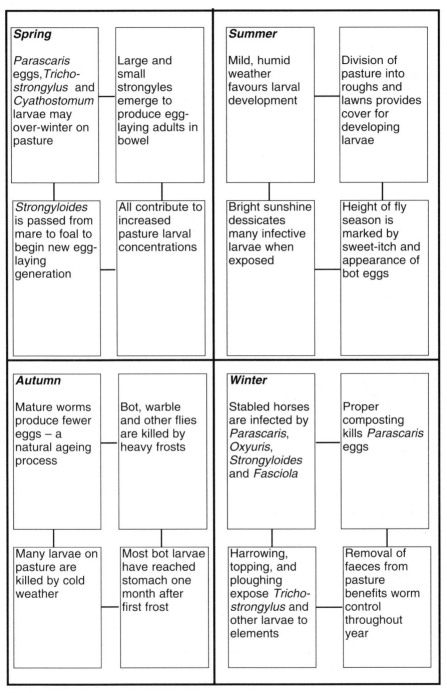

| Spring | | Summer | |
|---|---|---|---|
| *Parascaris* eggs, *Tricho-strongylus* and *Cyathostomum* larvae may over-winter on pasture | Large and small strongyles emerge to produce egg-laying adults in bowel | Mild, humid weather favours larval development | Division of pasture into roughs and lawns provides cover for developing larvae |
| *Strongyloides* is passed from mare to foal to begin new egg-laying generation | All contribute to increased pasture larval concentrations | Bright sunshine dessicates many infective larvae when exposed | Height of fly season is marked by sweet-itch and appearance of bot eggs |
| Autumn | | Winter | |
| Mature worms produce fewer eggs – a natural ageing process | Bot, warble and other flies are killed by heavy frosts | Stabled horses are infected by *Parascaris*, *Oxyuris*, *Strongyloides* and *Fasciola* | Proper composting kills *Parascaris* eggs |
| Many larvae on pasture are killed by cold weather | Most bot larvae have reached stomach one month after first frost | Harrowing, topping, and ploughing expose *Tricho-strongylus* and other larvae to elements | Removal of faeces from pasture benefits worm control throughout year |

*Problems through the year*

ufacturers of fenbendazole now recommend a five-day treatment course against encysted larvae.

Field trials have shown that conventional bi-monthly therapy with non-ivermectin drugs control large strongyles but not cyathostomes. Ivermectin suffers from the common failing that it does not kill encysted cyathostome larvae; however, it is effective against adults and against larvae that have emerged from the bowel wall and it does reduce the number of encysted larvae substantially. But encysted larvae are not removed, meaning that when horses are dosed and moved on they can still contaminate new pastures with this problem worm.

## Limiting Pasture Contamination

It is evident from the foregoing that earlier attitudes were deficient and that rationalisation must combine ideals of good pasture management with effective drug treatment. Erroneous thinking resulted in a loss of effectiveness of what were once excellent drugs. For the future, we must concentrate on limiting pasture build-up as well as treating horses at critical times, both to eliminate developed worm burdens as well as to prevent crises which may occur at particular times of the year.

It is now recommended that dosing twice, first in spring, then in summer, will help prevent seasonal rises in faecal egg counts, thereby limiting numbers of pasture larvae in summer and autumn. This advice applies particularly to northern latitudes, but the advice does not apply where there is limited grazing with heavy ground contamination, in which case more intensive anthelmintic programmes must be still maintained. In southern latitudes dosing on the same basis is carried out in the autumn and winter.

The spring rise in worm burdens occurs when environmental factors favour parasite infestation and this includes both external factors favouring larval development as well as the maturation to egg-laying of immature worms within the host. If this development is not checked, pasture contamination in summer and autumn will be maximal, with as many as 100,000 (or more) larvae per kilogramme of herbage being ingested in particularly intensive situations. It is also advised to treat for bots in the autumn and that drugs be alternated annually to prevent the development of resistance.

It should be appreciated, however, that animals with high faecal egg counts in the later months of the year are not creating exceptional problems because of the susceptibility of eggs and infective larvae to winter

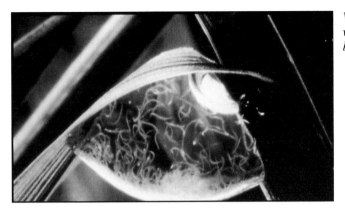

*Worm larvae in water droplet on blade of grass*

temperatures. Conversely, in warm southern latitudes, high temperatures destroy a large percentage of exposed infective larvae.

## Low-level Exposure

This type of approach does not eliminate all exposure to infective larvae. It has been noted that young horses are most severely affected by parasites and in these animals anthelmintic drugs are at their lowest level of efficiency. But some degree of exposure is considered desirable as a means of stimulating immunity; older animals exposed to worms for the first time may react with serious disease development.

Prevention means limiting exposure, an exercise which is unlikely ever to be totally effective, because of the nature of infection and the breadth of parasite species involved. But prevention is the essence of all good clinical medicine; the idea that disease can be lived with and treated with drugs when symptoms arise is a grave miscalculation. This kind of policy, relating to bacteria and viruses as well, is only ever likely to end in failure.

Prevention, in parasitic disease, means hygiene both within the stable and when at grass, the need to identify sources of contamination and aim to reduce or eliminate them. Pasture hygiene means, above all, limiting ground contamination, and this may well demand the physical removal of faeces, which is a duty that becomes vital in intensive situations.

## Pasture Hygiene

Plainly, grazing land does not become parasite infested without the presence of animals, and all pasture contamination is of faecal origin. This takes place either by direct soiling or indirectly through spreading of inadequately decomposed faeces onto grazing land.

Where possible, horses should not be kept on small, intensively-grazed paddocks because, as we know, parasite problems cannot be controlled by the effectiveness of anthelmintics alone. The best approach is in the judicious use of anthelmintic drugs coupled with intelligent pasture and stable hygiene. Good hygiene will reduce the need and frequency of drug use. And while faecal collection is not practicable where a small number of horses graze over large acreages, the greatest problems arise on intensively grazed paddocks and it is in the use of these that pasture hygiene and parasite control are of paramount importance. In these situations, horses are being exposed to huge numbers of eggs and larvae daily; anthelmintic use only influences developed and developing parasites within the host and have little influence on renewed intake. When it is appreciated that over 90 per cent of contamination can exist on the ground as opposed to within infected horses, the importance of hygiene becomes increasingly clear.

## Removing Faeces

To be effective, the removal of faeces from pasture should be carried out twice weekly, to prevent the dispersal of ascarid eggs and the development of infective strongyle larvae and their migration to vegetation. The possibility that cyathostomes develop to infectivity in two days under laboratory conditions is not thought relevant in field conditions.

Experiments in England during 1984, carried out at the Animal Health Trust at Newmarket, showed that this twice-weekly removal of faeces was more effective than routine treatment with anthelmintic drugs. Pasture contamination proved less than with drug-treated controls.

It has also been shown in the USA that yearlings, which are known to be more susceptible to parasites, benefit from pasture hygiene, as opposed to routine dosing, and are more likely to perform effectively as adults when this is provided. An added advantage of this approach is the effect of faecal removal on grazing habits: horses graze more intensively and pastures are not divided into bare areas and other rough sections which are not grazed at all, as normally occurs. Horses like clean grazing and large areas of available grazing are wasted through faecal contamination under most existing systems. Removal thus improves the economic production of a given pasture.

Other studies in the USA, in Ohio, have shown that contamination of the bare, grazed paddock areas with larvae can occur, especially as the grazing season progresses, and where animal numbers are high horses may be forced to graze the heavily contaminated rough areas in any case.

The problem of faecal removal is in the labour involved. While manual removal may be practical for small areas, mechanised cleaners are necessary for larger areas. And, while such equipment does exist, it is not widely available, but perhaps increasing horse numbers will alter this deficit in the future. Horse owners may well reject the idea because of the labour or expense involved, but the ultimate benefit, both financial and to animal health, makes it a serious proposition for the future.

## Harrowing and Topping

Harrowing, sometimes carried out on intensively grazed land, only helps to increase pasture contamination. While it may expose developing parasites to dessication in sunny conditions, it is a practice not to be recommended except perhaps where a pasture is to be rested and where prevailing conditions may reduce parasite numbers rather than make them more available to animals. Research in New Zealand indicated that foals grazing harrowed paddocks had heavier worm burdens than those on paddocks which were not.

Topping does not answer the problem either: greater concentrations of infective larvae are likely to exist closer to the soil surface.

## Resting

Resting pasture may allow developing larvae to die off, but this may take as long as a year to occur. Chemical control of larvae on pasture is not a feasible proposition either, due to cost, but there is also the influence added chemicals might have on our already heavily challenged environment.

## Mixed Grazing

Though mixed grazing can be effective for horses, both cattle and sheep, because of their different grazing habits, are necessary to reduce parasite exposure.

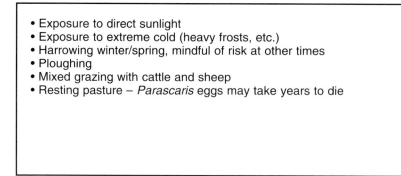

- Exposure to direct sunlight
- Exposure to extreme cold (heavy frosts, etc.)
- Harrowing winter/spring, mindful of risk at other times
- Ploughing
- Mixed grazing with cattle and sheep
- Resting pasture – *Parascaris* eggs may take years to die

*Factors favouring larval destruction*

Cattle tend to eat the upper vegetation, thus avoiding most equine parasites; sheep will crop the same pasture closer to the ground. Where cattle and sheep graze land until mid-summer and horses are then turned out on to it, most overwintered equine parasites should have been removed. Horses are then exposed to cattle and sheep parasites, of which *T. axei* is the most important species capable of infecting horses.

Therefore the practice of resting pastures, or systems of mixed grazing, are less practical than pasture hygiene because of weather-resistant worm stages, because of *T. axei* and because of cyathostomes.

Common sense must prevail in other areas too and horses sharing a pasture with donkeys are likely to become infected with lungworm.

## Dosing Reminders

To prevent build-up of infective larvae on pasture dosing in spring and summer is recommended. Pyrantel is effective against a range of adult large and small strongyles, ascarids, pinworms and tapeworms (at twice the normal dosage rate). It is not advocated as being effective against immature worms and its distinguishing capacity is its usefulness in dealing with tapeworms.

Fenbendazole is effective against a range of large and small strongyles but is the only drug claimed by manufacturers to be effective against the encysted larvae of cyathostomes; for this purpose a five-day treatment regime is advised. Ivermectin is effective against a wide range of adult and larval worm stages and it also reduces the problems caused by cyathostomes; its most commonly mentioned weakness is a lack of effectiveness against tapeworms at routine dosage rates. However it must be

- Natural spring rise due to emerging generation and winter survivors
- Intensity of grazing – number of horses per acre
- Failure to dose or use of ineffective drugs
- Warm, humid weather with good ground cover
- Heavily infected animals produce large numbers of eggs/larvae
- Transmission of *Strongyloides* larvae from mare to foal
- Transmission of *Parascaris* eggs from mare to foal
- Rough areas of pasture protect *Trichostrongylus* larvae
- Donkeys transmit lungworm
- Wet areas may harbour fluke
- Failure to remove bot eggs means certain infection

*Factors favouring larval build-up*

accepted that ivermectin is an excellent drug and its advent has added a new dimension to horse worming.

Ivermectin can be used at eight week intervals in adult horses because of its efficacy against larval stages (and suppression of egg-laying). Other anthelmintics require monthly use to ensure low pasture contamination.

Foaling mares may transmit *S. westeri* in their milk and this can be prevented by dosing on the day of foaling with ivermectin. Foals should thereafter be treated at eight weeks and then with their dams until weaning. A combination of piperazine and thiabendazole in the past was effective in dealing with routine encountered burdens in the first six months of life.

Some authorities advise that drugs should be rotated annually so that each generation of worms is exposed to one drug only, but there is a dearth of scientific evidence to support this when using ivermectin; it applies mainly to benzimidazoles.

Pinworms, stomach worms and those that cause summer sores and cutaneous onchocerciasis are of lesser significance at a herd level than other roundworms encountered. These will require individual treatment as will the growing nuisance of tapeworms.

Faecal egg counts taken at critical times, like spring and summer, will indicate burdens before and after treatment and an effective drug should keep egg counts at below 100 eggs per gram of faeces between treatments. Where these increase greatly, it may well be advised to move animals onto clean pastures when dosed.

The whole idea of a dosing routine is to reduce worm burdens carried by grazing animals and thus limit pasture contamination. This ideal is greatly helped by thoughtful pasture hygiene which should ultimately reduce drug use. Where it is possible to implement faecal removal,

---

- *Oxyuris*
- *Parascaris*
- Bots
- Liver fluke (contaminated hay)
- *Strongyloides* (mare to foal, etc.)
- Tapeworm (through the intermediate host)

---

*Parasites of horses kept in stables or in open barns*

treatments can be reduced, grazing areas increased and supplementary feeding may be avoided.

After weaning the main threat of pasture contamination comes from cyathostomes, migrating ascarids and large strongyles. On heavily-infested pastures, infective strongyle larvae could well persist until the following spring, as well as ascarid eggs (though immunity here usually develops after about six months of age). The emerging generation of encysted cyathostomes help to contaminate spring pastures and the possibility of *T. axei* occurring at this time should not be overlooked.

The benefits of such a system arise from greater parasite control without heavy drug requirements; more effective pasture use and greater productivity; less risk of drug resistance; and less drug cost.

## Vital Points

1. The degree of intensification is decided by the amount of grass available, the number of horses and the presence of other species grazing the same land. Inevitably, a farmer with hundreds of hectares is in a different position from a small owner with a paddock that is heavily grazed, possibly worm sick and with no alternative source of grass or exercise. In the latter case, pasture hygiene is vital and worming routines need to be carefully considered.
2. Season is important as climate not only affects parasite development but by various means influences the availability of infective worms to grazing animals.
3. The cleanest grass is new pasture, after the plough, but the possiblity exists of the development of some eggs which have contaminated the ground prior to ploughing.

4. Lower intake of infective parasites helps overall control as well as reducing the risk of drug resistance.

## Stable Hygiene

Hygiene in stabling regimes is as important to the control of some parasites as it is to other infectious conditions which may thrive in dirt. This means frequent sterilisation of all exposed surfaces, either chemically, by pressure hose or steam-cleaning. It also means consideration of food sources where these might carry disease.

Not only may encysted metacercariae of liver fluke be present in hay, but eggs of worms like *Parascaris* may develop and become infective within the stable. The pinworm, *Oxyuris*, may adhere to surfaces which are accessible to it.

Also, fly habitats are often created by poor hygiene. Thus, decaying organic matter, like dung, traces of food, unclean containers and their like, may foster disease in both direct and indirect ways.

The answer to liver fluke in hay is to be certain of the source of the hay and to avoid any that comes from suspect pasture. However, this may be virtually impossible when buying hay or silage from a dealer.

## Control Routines

For owners of small or intensive paddocks, the following routine should be observed in order to maintain hygiene and promote general efficiency:
—carry out regular faecal examination or laboratory tests;
—regularly remove faeces;
—dose animals before turnout and bi-monthly thereafter;
—dose with ivermectin or, monthly, with other drugs;
—rest paddocks wherever possible;
—rotate paddocks with sheep or cattle to lower exposure for horses;
—remember precautions surrounding *T. axei*.

## Practical Aspects of Worming

The practical side of treating horses for worms is relatively uncomplicated for today's horse owner. There is a limited number of drugs available, most of which are given either as a paste directly into the horse's mouth or as a powder or granules which are added to the feed. However, the quality of available drugs means that, within certain limitations, each product has its own part to play in the general scheme of worm treatment, prevention and control.

Most of these anthelminthic drugs are now available through veterinary surgeons, chemists, merchants, saddlers, tack shops and so on. The critical factor in availability is that the drugs are registered as PML (Pharmacists and Merchants List Category) drugs in law and available only from merchants and saddlers on the basis that there are qualified persons engaged in their sale. The training for obtaining such a qualification is subject to courses provided by the Animal Medicines Training Regulatory Authority (AMTRA). In the case of saddlers, the qualification means that an individual responsible for the storage, sale and supply of PML horse wormers has a knowledge of anatomy and physiology, husbandry and nutrition as well as diseases of the horse and the laws that govern the sale of these products. Such an individual will hold a certificate issued by AMTRA and will be entered on the list of Suitably Qualified Persons (SQP) compiled by that organisation.

Licences to sell these products are issued by the Royal Pharmaceutical Society (Animal Medicines Division) whose authority is dervived from the Medicines Act (1968), the particular instrument being the Medicines (Veterinary Drugs Pharmacy and Merchants' List) Order 1992.

Saddlers and tack shops are included under what is described as the Saddlers List; their premises are required to be registered with the Royal Pharmaceutical Society and they are obliged to engage a member of staff who holds the AMTRA certificate.

## Worming Procedures

Most horses accept oral pastes without great difficulty, the biggest problem being where parts of the dose are lost by falling from the horse's mouth. An applicator is slipped through the interdental space between the incisor and molar teeth and the paste deposited on the base of the tongue. It is usual to hold the animal's head up as it swallows to prevent loss of drug. Naturally, where a portion of the dose is lost, the shortfall must be replaced, otherwise the treatment will not be effective.

These pastes are usually contained in graded applicators, and a measured dose is easily given which will relate to the age and weight of the horse. It is not normally necessary to withold feed prior to dosing.

An important procedure to keep in mind here is the handling of syringes. It is common for all syringes that contain anthelmintic pastes to contain a locking device that can be adjusted along the barrel of the syringe in order to grade the dosage for animals which (due to age or weight) are not given a full syringe. Care *must* be taken to ensure that this mechanism is operated effectively to prevent overdosage and it is also important to store unused or partly-used syringes in a cool dark place with their caps replaced after administration.

Weight may be measured on a weighing scales, but it is often calculated on the basis of size and development by individuals experienced in these matters. However, while there is normally a margin of safety, and multiple doses are recommended in particular worm infections, it is critical to adhere to the manufacturer's advised dosages in all cases. It is also necessary to be aware of any contra-indications for use – for example, pregnancy, age, illness and so on.

With horses or ponies that prove impossible to dose in this way, the same drugs can often be given using a powder that can be contained in the food; and where animals are reluctant to eat the powder, the option remains to hide the drug by coating it with molassess, and so on – or, if all else fails, it may be administered by stomach tube.

Again, two important points need to be noted here: first, the use of a stomach tube should *only* be carried out by an experienced veterinary surgeon as it is a *highly dangerous exercise* for anyone without training; secondly, it has been known for liquid or injectable anthelmintics to be given which are not licensed for use in horses and it must be appreciated that anyone who follows such a policy is taking a *risk* with their animal's safety as well as having no comeback if anything were to go wrong.

Larvicidal drugs are those that kill helminth parasites in their larval stages. While it has always been suggested that there may be some risk in killing larvae that have found their way into blood vessels, this is not a general experience today, although there can be reactions. Horses carrying heavy burdens of *Onchocerca* microfilariae may deveop oedema and pruritis for a few days after treatment with ivermectin, but this is not considered serious and the symptoms usually pass off without treatment.

## Specific Drugs

The following information is given in alphabetical order and is *not* an indication of the relative importance of each drug.

The reader is therefore advised that, when using any drug, the manufacturers' directions must be followed and particular care should be taken to read the warnings and contra-indications for their use. The list is generally confined to drugs presently available.

### Carbon disulphide

A highly-volatile foul-smelling liquid, used in the past for the removal of bots from horses. Usually given by stomach tube to horses which had been fasted, it has today largely been replaced by safer, more affective and more easily administered drugs.

### Dichlorvos

An organophosphorus anthelminthic and insecticide used in horses mainly for bot removal, but which also removes a range of other parasites. No longer marketed for use in horses in the United Kingdom and Ireland.

### Febantel (Bayverm)

A benzimidazole drug available in pelletted form for horses. Febantel is closely related to fenbendazole and oxfendazole. It is given at a dose rate of 6 mg febental/kg bodyweight (equal to 32g of pellets per 100kg).

Febantel is recommended for use against benzimidazole-susceptible strains of large and small strongyles, ascarids, and *Oxyuris*.

### Fenbendazole (Panacur)

A benzimidazole drug available as granules, paste, or in suspension. In horses it is effective against large and small strongyles, ascarids, *Oxyuris*, and *Strongyloides*. This drug has been found effective against the larval stages of *Cyathostomum* when encysted in the wall of the intestine and it is used for this purpose on a five-day treatment basis; this is advised as best being done in late October or early November, but the manufacturer advises its use to the end of the year.

Fenbendazole is also effective against immature and migrating strongyle larvae.

Panacur 10 per cent suspension is used at a rate of 1ml per 13kg bodyweight (equal to 7.5mg fenbendazole/kg bodyweight). For the treatment of mucosal stages of small strongyles it is used at four times the standard dose rate. For the treatment of migrating large strongyles it is used at eight times the standard dose rate. For the treatment of migrating large strongyles and the mucosal stages of small strongyles, 3.75ml of suspension per 50kg bodyweight is given daily for five days (equal to 7.5mg/kg bodyweight daily). This dose can be given in the feed and works out at 45ml daily for a horse weighing 600kg.

For the treatment of *Strongyloides* in three-week old suckling foals a dose of 25ml per 50kg/bodyweight is given.

Panacur 22 per cent granules may be used for exactly the same purposes and the preparation is recommended at a standard dose rate of 5g per 150kg/bodyweight, and *pro rata*, mixed in the feed.

This drug is safe to use in pregnant mares and in foals and no dietary control is required either before or after treatment with Panacur paste, which is contained in a syringe, the full contents of which provide a standard dose for a 500kg horse.

As before, the dose rates of paste are *pro rata* for the conditions specified above; for foals with *Strongyloides* a full syringe per 75kg/bodyweight is given.

## Haloxon (Multiwurma)

An organophosphorus drug available as a white powder containing 15.3g haloxon per 25g powder. The powder is used on foals over two months old and adult horses and is useful against large and small strongyles, *Oxyuris* and bots. It is given mixed in the normal feed.

The recommended dose rate is 25g of powder to a foal over two months old or for a pony up to 300kg. Twice this amount is given to medium-sized hunters, Thoroughbreds and so on, or three times the amount to heavyweights.

Among the contra-indications for use are: do not dose foals younger than two months old; do not dose mares in the first four weeks of pregnancy. This product is toxic to geese and it is advised that these birds do not get access to the faeces of treated horses. The drug should not be combined with any other organophosphorus-containing drug, or be used on any horse within seven days of previous use. Be careful of using on sick or convalescent animals.

There are no side effects when the drug is used as advised, but over-dosage is dangerous, especially in older animals.

## Ivermectin (Eqvalan)

Available as a paste for horses given at a dosage rate of 0.2mg/kg body-weight of active principle.

Ivermectin is a broad-spectrum anhelminthic with a wide range of activity against adult and larval stages of worms at standard dose rates. It has been found safe for use in foals, broodmares and stallions.

The drug is effective against the adult and larval stages of both large and small strongyles and there is a suppression of egg-laying for up to ten weeks after treatment. This means that ivermectin is safe to use at two-month intervals, where other drugs may need to be used more frequently. However, it is not fully effective against the encysted stage of *Cyathostomum* species but work carried out in Warwick in 1993 suggests a significant (up to 77 per cent) reduction in the development of encysted larvae within the wall of the bowel when ivermectin is used.

The drug is highly effective gainst larvae within the lumen of the bowel.

Ivermectin is also effective against adult and immature lungworms, *Oxyuris*, ascarids; adult *Trichostrongylus*, *Habronema*, and *Strongyloides*; microfilariae of *Onchocerca*; and the oral and gastric stages of bots. Ivermectin is not effective against tapeworms. A single syringe will dose a 600kg horse.

The only warning given with ivermectin is the possibility of reactions where animals are suffering from heavy burdens of *Onchocerca* microfilariae. These may be oedema and puritis, but the symptoms generally resolve in a few days.

### Levamisole

Not commonly used today for horses. Available as Nilverm, in liquid form, it is not licensed for use in horses, but is sometimes used in combination with drugs like piperazine and given by stomach tube. It has a narrow margin of safety for horses and a low efficacy against equine parasites.

### Mebendazole (Telmin)

A benzimidazole drug available as white granules or paste, the granules containing 100mg/g of active principle, the paste containing a total of 4g active principle per syringe.

Mebendazole is a broad-spectrum anthelminthic recommended for use in the horse an donkey, active against large and small strongyles, ascarids, *Oxyuris*, lungworm, *Trichostrongylus*. It is sometimes combined with trichlorfon to combat bots as well. It is a very safe drug for use in horses and is used at a rate of 5–10mg/kg bodyweight. Foals over six weeks old are given half the contents of a syringe; horses and ponies up to 544kg, a full syringe; heavy hunters, one-and-a-half syringes; and horses over 680kg, two syringes. Using the granules, which come in sachets containing 2g mebendazole, the dose varies from half a sachet for foals over six weeks to two sachets for horses over 272kg.

### Oxfendazole (Systamex, Synanthic)

A benzimidazole drug not licenced for use in horses in the United

Kingdom at present. It has a similar range of activity to that of mebendazole.

### Oxibendazole (Equidin, Equitac, Lincoln Horse and Pony Wormer Paste)

Comes as a paste, and has a similar range of activity to that of other benzimidazole drugs. It is recommended for use against large and small strongyles, ascarids, *Oxyuris* and *Strongyloides* (where it is used at one-and-a-half times the standard dose). The normal dose rate is 10mg/kg bodyweight (15mg/kg for *Strongyloides*), the contents of one syringe being adequate to dose a horse of 500kg.

Oxibendazole is used on foals over six weeks old and is safe in pregnant mares and working stallions. It has no effect against bots.

### Oxyclozanide (Zanil)

Not licensed for use in horses, oxyclozanide is used as the drug of choice for liver fluke in this species. A maximum dose of 100ml is given to an adult horse.

Care needs to be taken in using this product and it should not be used in conjunction with any other drug. Its effect is to kill adult fluke in the bile ducts and it is not claimed to have any effect on immature fluke within the substance of the liver.

### Piperazine

A commonly-used drug in the past, especially for treatment of ascariasis in foals, piperazine was also found to be effective against some large and small strongyles. At a dosage rate of 110mg/kg bodyweight, it was used in foals at about eight weeks and could be repeated at monthly intervals thereafter.

Piperazine was commonly administered by stomach tube in conjunction with thiabendazole or other benzimidazole drugs. It has largely been superceded by drugs which are easier to administer and are effective against a wider spectrum of parasites.

### Pyrantel embonate (Strongid-P)

Available as a paste or as granules. It is effective against adult large and small strongyles, *Oxyuris*, ascarids, and tapeworm (at an increased dosage rate).

The granules are safe and palatble and can be given in the animal's feed or administered by stomach tube, and are recommended for use in foals over four weeks old. There is no need to withhold food prior to dosing, but any animal is more likely to consume the full of its dose if hungry when fed.

Used at a dosage rate of 19mg pyrantel/kg bodyweight, a sachet of granules contains 5.18g of pyrantel embonate, enough to dose a horse of 137kg bodyweight. For tapewrom, twice this dosage is used. If using the loose granules, one level measure, supplied by the manufacturer, is used per 45kg bodyweight.

Pyrantel is safe in foals over four weeks old, in working stallions and in-foal mares as long as the recommended dosing rates are followed.

The paste is contained in a syringe the contents of which will dose one horse of 550kg bodyweight. Foals and other animals up to 275kg bodyweight receive half a syringe.

It is advised to use this drug at four to six week intervals in summer and autumn. Foals are dosed at one month and thereafter at four-week intervals; mares are dosed at three to four days before turning out and suckler mares dosed at four-week intervals thereafter.

Where tapeworm is being treated, any need for retreatment should be carried out six weeks after the initial treatment.

**Trichlorfon**
An organic compound used in the past for the removal from horses of bots, ascarids, and *Oxyuris*. It is no longer an element of routine worming programmes.

## Worming Calendar

The level of infection will, of course, be gauged by the degree of intensification, body condition of foals, worm counts, and so on. However, horse owners could adopt the following programme, and worm:

—all horses prior to spring turnout;
—broodmares two to three days before foaling;
—foals for *Strongyloides*, at two to three weeks old but only in intensive conditions or where there is evidence of infection;
—foals at one to two months, for *Parascaris* and regularly thereafter depending on efficacy of drug and advised frequency of treatment;
—April/May, to prevent a build up of larvae in spring;
—July, to contain high level of larvae expected in summer in intensive situations;

—end of August, in intensive situations;

—for bots, three weeks after the last frost;

—October/November, for tapeworms and six weeks later if a repeat dose is required; also ten weeks after spring turnout in intensive situations;

—October/December, for migrating strongyles and encysted small strongyles;

—horses kept indoors when they come in and one or two months thereafter to remove developing larvae.

If using benzimidazole drugs, horses should be dosed during the grazing season every four to six weeks, remembering resistance as a factor in small strongyles.

Dose with ivermectin, every eight weeks if required.

And dose at four to six weeks using pyrantel.

## Insecticides

These are marketed in varying forms and using a number of proprietary names. Some of those insecticides more commonly encountered are discussed below.

**Coumaphos (contained in Negasunt)**
An organophosphorus compound which is applied to wounds to prevent attack by flies or to kill larvae that may have hatched from their eggs.

**Benzyl Benzoate (at 25 per cent, contained in Sweet Itch Plus)**
A clear, oily liquid used as a topical application for most external parasites. It has no residual effect, therefore must be applied repeatedly. It is commonly used in sweet itch in horses where it is seen to provide a degree of relief in some cases.

**Cypermethrin (at 5 per cent, contained in Barricade and Deosan Deosect)**
A residual insecticide for use in horses against flies and lice; used as a 5 per cent solution or a concentrate to which water is added (follow manufacturers' instructions). It is a synthetic product similar to pyrethrum. For general fly control it is advised to use at the beginning of the fly season and every two to four weeks thereafter depending on the level of infestation.

For lice, apply once infestation is noted and repeat at not less than two week intervals.

### Piperonyl Butoxide and Pyrethrum (contained in Dermoline, Extra Tail, Sweet Itch Lotion)

These are synergistic drugs, available as a spray, shampoo or lotion. They are used to kill and repel flies and are also effective against lice. Do not allow these drugs to come in contact with eyes or mucous membranes. Follow manufacturers' instructions for application. For lice, ensure the shampoo remains in contact with the animal for at least ten minutes. Also take steps to prevent reinfestation by treating blankets, tack, grooming equipment and all contact surfaces.

The preparation is non-toxic and safe to use in all horses.

### Permethrin (in Switch, Fly-Repellent Plus, Lincoln Lice Control Plus)

A synthetic product similar to pyrethrum. It is available in solution (Switch) for the treatment and control of sweet itch. With a maximum dose rate of 40ml, it is used at a rate of 1ml per 10kg bodyweight, applying the measured dose along the horse's back including the mane and rump.

Treatment is advised on a weekly basis but may be required more frequently in bad cases.

Warning is given of a possible adverse reaction in fine-skinned horses.

## Antifungals

As with the insecticides, antifungals too are available in a variety of forms and names. Again, not all can be mentioned here, but the following are a good cross-section.

### Griseofulvin (Fulcin, Dufulvin, Equifulvin, Grisol, Norofulvin)

An antifungal antibiotic effective against ringworm caused by *Trichophyton* and *Microsporum* species.

Available as a powder, granules or paste, the drug is administered for seven consecutive days and the dosage varies with the product used. However, the recommended dose of griseofulvin is 7.5mg/kg bodyweight daily, usually provided at the rate of 20g of powder/granules per 150kg bodyweight daily (but read manufacturers' literature). The powder form is normally consumed in the feed without protest, but in some cases it may be necessary to add molasses to improve accceptability. The dosage of paste is the same but computed by the strength of the product and the size of the syringe in which it is contained.

There is no effect against systemic fungal infections, and the drug is not advised for use in pregnant mares. There is also a warning against prolonged treatment because of experience in other species.

In treating ringworm of horses it is important to appreciate the infectious nature of the condition and disinfect tack, equipment, and all contact surfaces.

### Enilconazole (Imaverol and Miconazole)

A synthetic antifungal available as an oily liquid which is effective against *Trichophyton* and *Microsporum* species.

The liquid is diluted one part in 50 parts of water in which it emulsifies and is applied topically. Crusts should be removed using a hard brush (which should be dipped in the emulsion before and after use). If the extent of the condition is extensive, the whole animal should be treated; if the lesions are fairly localised, treat all lesions and the surrounding area. Repeat the treatment for four times, at three-day intervals.

### Natamycin (Mycophyt)

A topical antifungal powder which is used as a suspension in water (adding 2 litres of water to Mycophyt 2, or 10 litres to Mycophyt 10). The suspension is applied directly or sprayed onto the affected area, or the whole animal (depending on the extent of infection). Treatment may be repeated if required some four to five days later. It is advised not to expose treated animals to direct sunlight on the day of treatment, nor to use in conjunction with other topical applications. The drug may not be effective on skin which has been treated with any greasy application in previous days.

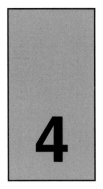

# 4 Laboratory Procedures

## Diagnosis

The clinical signs produced by internal parasites will depend to a great extent on the identity and nature of the predominant parasite, on the kind of tissue damage it creates, and on the burden of worms within the host. Thus with small burdens of even important worms the external signs may be negligible, although the effect on the individual animal may hold serious consequences for, say, horses in training.

The principle diagnostic monitor of low-level worm infections is the examination of faeces in the laboratory. By this procedure worm eggs and larvae are identified and counted so that approximate information can be had of burdens being carried and this also provides indications as to likely herbage contamination, taking into consideration details of season, animal numbers, paddock size, and so on.

It would be wrong to imagine that laboratory examination is flawless, or that results provide all the information we might desire. The small strongyle, *Cyathostomum*, at one stage of development, becomes encysted in the bowel wall, at which point it is non-egg-laying and extremely resistant to drugs used in routine worm dosing. Faecal worm counts can give no indication of this situation.

The gross clinical signs of these conditions may be indicative of the cause in certain cases. For example, pot-bellied foals that are unthrifty and kept in intensive or semi-intensive conditions are very likely to be carrying roundworms. However, this is not a positive diagnosis – which can only be confirmed by either faecal or post-mortem examination. Other symptoms, like anaemia, oedema, diarrhoea, are all non-specific disease signs and cannot on their own do anything more than suggest a diagnosis in conjunction with details of history and the like – and, very often, response to treatment. Laboratory examination of blood helps, to some extent, to extend this picture. However, very few tests except for direct tissue examinations provide specific results useful in diagnosis; all of which must impress on the reader the need for constructive attitudes to parasite treatment and control.

Where horses are kept intensively, a positive approach is essential, and when horses in small numbers graze limited, bare paddocks, the dangers need to be recognised. The term 'horse-sick' in relation to grazing is not a misnomer nowadays. Anthelmintic (wormer) drugs on their own are unable to prevent this from happening.

## Faecal Examination

When parasites inhabiting the digestive tract are traced through examination of the faeces at a laboratory it is not always possible to determine their clinical significance. These samples are usually submitted through the local veterinary practice, who will advise on treatment, depending on results. Large studfarms may have their own laboratory and will engage trained personnel to carry out faecal and other tests.

Collection of fresh faecal samples and their later submission to special techniques exposes the presence of eggs, larvae or cysts within them. However, a negative result is not always significant; adult lungworm, for example, do not always succeed in reproducing in horses (not being the natural host) and the bot-fly pupa also does not emerge (except at a particular time of the year). So, again, negative faecal findings in these instances could hide a high worm burden. And so too with liver fluke which, in any case, are intermittent egg-layers: negative results in relation to this parasite may prove misleading.

Many parasitic forms have a characteristic morphology (shape) and are easily recognised in the laboratory. But some eggs of nematodes, flukes or tapeworms cannot be distinguished individually in this way. This is not necessarily a problem as the presence of large numbers of unspecified worm eggs might only cause concern if the worm involved proved resistant to treatment. Specific identification is generally a matter for a specialist laboratory.

Mange or scab mites also appear in faeces as a result of being licked from the skin and may have no significance when found there. Pollen grains, plant hairs, grain mites, mould spores and plant and animal debris also appear in faeces. Parasite eggs or cysts from one species may be found in the gut of another. The clinical significance of these might be considered in the light of symptoms and the presence or absence of other parasites.

## Materials

Fresh faecal samples are collected direct from the stable or paddock and placed in a 60g screw-topped jar. If sent by post, they must be placed in a leak-proof container. Taking samples from stale faeces which has been voided for unknown periods may only lead to false results.

Laboratory examination involves, first, mixing the faeces with a flotation fluid – a liquid with a specific gravity greater than that of, for example, eggs, but less than the specific gravity of the faecal debris. The parasite forms thus rise to the top of the fluid when suspended in it. The most common flotation solutions include heavy concentrations of sodium chloride, sucrose (cane or beet sugar), glycerine, zinc sulphate, zinc acetate, sodium nitrate, sodium acetate or magnesium sulphate; but none are ideal. Glycerine has too high a viscosity; saline solutions are low in viscosity but tend to dehydrate and distort parasitic forms; they also crystallise quickly on the micro-slide thus preventing proper examination of the sample. Solutions of high specific gravity will float too much debris, thus defeating the purpose in a different way.

Heavy or granulated sugar (sucrose) has a specific gravity of 1.200 to 1.300 and is found to be one of the best materials available. However, it fails to float most tapeworm eggs, flukes and thorny headed worms. A centrifuge capable of revolving at 1,500rpm should be used and the make up of the flotation solution should be:

–granulated sugar 454gm
–tap water 355ml
–40 per cent formaldehyde solution 6ml.

The microscope lens, mirrors and objective, eye pieces and substage condenser must all be kept free of dust and other foreign matter. Microscope magnifications of 80 to 100 low power and 344 to 430 high power are best for faecal examinations. A mechanical stage and binocular body tube save time and eye strain. An oil immersion objective is an added asset for more detailed work.

## Procedure

A number of steps need to be taken and in the correct sequence, as:

1. The faecal sample should be moist. If not, add water to soften it and make a semi-solid suspension.
2. Add between 1gm and 2gm of faeces to a paper cup.
3. Add 15ml of flotation solution.
4. Stir until faeces are thoroughly suspended.
5. Strain into a test tube, using something like a tongue depressor to press out most of the liquid.
6. Centrifuge at 1,500rpm for three minutes. (The sample could also be allowed to sit for a few hours for flotation to occur.)
7. Transfer a drop from the top of the column to a slide and cover with a coverglass.
8. Place under the microscope. The slide is then scanned using a 50X or 100X magnification and the field is examined methodically for the presence of eggs, larvae, and so on.

## Alternative Procedure

A modification of the same method is used for fluke eggs. An alternative method, sometimes used in practice laboratories, is to smear a light coating of faeces onto a slide and examine it directly under a microscope. While the procedure has its limitations it is useful for the detection of nematode larvae and some protozoa. The coating of the material on the slide, however, needs to be sufficiently thin to allow differentiation of the objects being examined.

The routine examination of faeces for evidence of parasitism is not an unduly difficult task. It could be undertaken by a lay person, assuming he or she possessed the correct equipment and had been trained beforehand by a laboratory technician or veterinary surgeon. However, any such person would need to recognise their own limitations and seek advice when in doubt.

It should be appreciated, too, that counting worm eggs is not an exact procedure, but is a very good guide to current worm burdens. While different results may arise from samples taken from the same dropping, readings above 100 eggs per gram of faeces are generally considered significant.

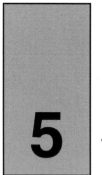

# 5  The Skin

The skin is the largest body organ and it varies in thickness over various parts; it has been estimated in man that skin accounts for in the region of 15 per cent of body weight.

In horses, wherever danger of injury is greatest the skin is correspondingly thick. Hence the skin covering the back, loins, quarters and limbs is thickest; that covering the face, muzzle, flanks, and inner side of the limbs, feels paper thin to handle. Yet, even the thinnest skin possesses great tensile strength.

The skin is least thick in the Thoroughbred and Arab, and thickest in the draught breeds. The thickness in ponies tends to vary according to whether they retain their true type or have been crossed with Thoroughbreds.

## Anatomy and Purpose

The skin consists of two principal layers, the superficial epidermis and the deeper dermis. Sensory nerves, blood vessels and glands (both sweat and sebaceous) are present in the dermis. The epidermis is without blood vessels and its outer layers are formed by dying and dead cells (the stratum corneum), which eventually are cast off (desquamate). The deepest epidermal layer (the stratum germinativum), is responsible for regeneration to compensate for this loss. This layer also contains melanin, a black or brown pigment which absorbs ultraviolet radiation and protects the skin and body from the effects of excessive sunlight. The epidermis is perforated by the passage of hairs and their follicles and by the ducts of glands.

The principal purpose of skin is to prevent penetration of liquids and noxious gases into the body, and this is aided by fatty secretions from sebaceous glands onto its surface. An equally important function is temperature regulation, aided by the hairs and sweat glands. Sensory perception (through the sense of touch) is controlled through the skin and some areas are more sensitive than others in this regard. Parts such as the lips and muzzle are provided with long feeler hairs which are connected to sensitive roots of associated sensory nerves. Horses use these especially when feeding both from the ground and from a manger. Mares nuzzle their foals with them and it is possible they recognise their offspring in this way, as well as by sound and the sense of smell.

## Skin Musculature

The skin is attached to the underlying parts of the horse's body by the subcutaneous connective tissue containing elastic fibres and fat, the subcutis.

In some parts of the body, notably the neck and back, tenseness is maintained by the presence in the subcutis of a thin voluntary muscle layer, the cutaneous muscle, intimately adherent to the skin. This muscle has only a limited attachment to the skeleton: the part in the neck attaches to the front of the sternum; the abdominal layer covers a large part of the

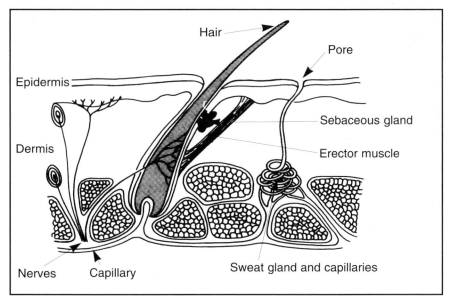

*Section through skin*

body behind the shoulder and arm, and has attachments to the humerus in front and the patella above the stifle at the back. On contraction it can twitch the skin and rid the greater part of the body of flies, dust, dirt and other irritants. By being adherent to the skin the cutaneous muscle may create shivering by very rapid contractions; this raises the local temperature by bringing warm blood to the cold surface. In a few places, notably the face, the cutaneous muscle is modified and the skin is less adherent to it.

## Skin Glands

The skin glands consist of sebaceous and sweat glands. The sebaceous glands produce sebum while the sweat glands, of course, produce sweat. The sebaceous glands are minute structures freely distributed throughout the whole of the horse's skin in close association with the hair roots.

## Sebum

Sebum is not a true secretion but a waxy material, consisting of cholesterol and waxes, which renders the skin pliable and waterproof; it contains substances which are converted into vitamin D by the action of sunlight.

Spread thinly over the individual hairs, sebum is responsible for the gloss of the coat; this is enhanced by regular grooming. Sebum also helps to give water resistance to the skin surface. However, it is suggested that overproduction of sebum is the basis of acne.

## Sweat

Sweat is one of the most dilute body fluids, the main purpose of which is the control of body temperature. Horse sweat is rich in electrolytes and contains as much as 15g per litre of protein, which allows for more effective evaporation. The horse is one of the few hairy animals in which sweating occurs over almost the whole body surface, the exception being the legs. Sweating is a continuous process and normally evaporation takes place, except during the fastest gaits, as rapidly as sweat is produced.

It has been estimated that the sweat secretion of a horse grazing out of doors in ordinary summer weather and choosing its own pace averages about 7kg of fluid in 24 hours without visible dampening of the body surface. When galloped, the resulting loss of fluid is inevitably much greater; perhaps twice the amount in a single hour.

Sweating is influenced by external temperature, humidity, length of coat, excitement, environment, work, and pace. A horse may sweat, however, when it is hot or cold. In the latter case sweating arises from nervous stimulation causing release of adrenalin into the blood which stimulates particular areas of the brain. It is often this effect, caused by anxiety, which makes a horse sweat prior to a race, even on a cold day. However, it is also a known side-effect in animals suffering from some virus infections.

Horses that sweat too freely lose weight. This is partly due to fluid loss from the blood and tissues – mainly water content – and this situation tends to be aggravated by the resulting disturbance of electrolytes within the body systems.

## Hair

Hair covers practically the entire body surface. However, more hair is carried over the parts of the skin exposed to direct sunlight than on the less exposed areas such as the inner surface of the ears, the inner side of the thighs, the perinaeum and the external genitalia in both sexes.

The skin carries permanent hair in the mane and tail, in the feather of some heavy breeds and in the eyelashes and long hairs of the muzzle. Permanent hair goes on growing indefinitely regardless of the temperature changes. The bulk of the hair covering the body is temporary hair, however, which is shed and changed for a new growth in spring and autumn, in preparation for the summer and winter coats. This temporary hair consists of closely placed patches of long hairs, some four to five per square centimetre which tend to hide the undercoat from view. This undercoat is made up of densely packed finer and shorter hairs, as many as 650 per square centimetre of skin.

Hair plays an important role in temperature regulation. Skin is a poor conductor of heat, especially when left ungroomed and dirty. This is why horses being roughed off are not brushed and encouraged to grow long coats by having their rugs left off. Hair responds in automatic fashion to heat and cold. In a cold atmosphere the hairs tend to rise and form a blanket imprisoning a layer of warm air. In warm weather the coat lies flat, but the skin may be cooled by the evaporation of sweat from its surface. The rise and fall of hair is due partly to the action of cutaneous muscle beneath the skin, but mainly to the reflexes of tiny involuntary muscle fibres attached to each hair follicle in the dermis. In the horse, hair raising is activated by cold but not by fear or anger – as in the cat and dog, and occasional human!

The deciding factor in coat casting is temperature, but the number of hours of daylight is also important in this. If horses are kept under artificial light and heat in winter – as mares are frequently in order to induce early ovulation – they soon start shedding heavy coats no matter how low the temperature is outside. Similarly, in cold conditions the coat grows rapidly and to a greater length. As a rule the new coat is growing underneath the old and tends to push the latter off.

Hard conditions delay coat casting, while good feeding and the provision of oils and essential vitamins will hasten the process. Mares shabby in coat can be slow to conceive and many fail to produce fertile ovarian follicles until the new coat has made its appearance.

Crossing indigenous ponies with Thoroughbreds or Arabs produces a change in the type of coat. Such animals are less able to withstand winter conditions on moors and hills.

## Functions of Skin

1. Mechanical protection from physical injury, including burns.
2. Protection from poisonous substances, microorganisms, and so on.
3. To prevent the loss of essential fluids and chemicals (thus preventing dehydration).
4. To assist in the control of body temperature.
5. Adaptation to external stimuli through responses to heat and cold.
6. Communication with the environment through the sense of touch.
7. Responses to physical insult through the sensation of pain.
8. Secretion of sweat and sebum and also the excretion of some waste products.
9. Protection against irradiation.
10. Production of vitamin D.
11. Plays a part in the immune system.
12. Responsible for production of the hooves – and organs like the eyes and the mammary glands.

## Diagnosis of Skin Disease

The diagnosis of skin disease is based firstly on visual examination of lesions followed by laboratory examination of scrapings and biopsies and so on. In examining lesions, the difference in type of skin reaction is important. For example: if there are fluid filled or hard bumps; if there is thickening of the skin; circumscribed areas; changes of pigmentation and so on. The size, distribution and nature of lesions all have an important bearing, and it is also of concern whether or not the animal shows signs of irritation and to what extent this is manifested if present.

Vesicles are small fluid filled structures – blisters. Pustules contain pus. Erosions only involve the epidermis, while ulcers are deeper in nature. Alopecia is loss of hair.

## Laboratory Investigation

Skin scrapings are the most common investigative sample taken for skin conditions. This is essentially a task for the veterinarian as it is quite easy to take too little or too much skin, making the sample useless in the former case, and causing unnecessary harm to the animal in the latter.

The sample so taken may be transferred straight onto a microscope slide and examined as it stands for the presence of parasites and fungi. However, negative results may arise in cases where a parasite has not appeared in the examined sample and it is wise to take the scraping from more than one lesion in order to increase the chances of success.

Samples containing pus may be cultured for bacteria and sensitivity tests carried out for guidance on treatment. However, it must be appreciated that organisms present may not be the cause of the skin condition seen and use of treatment in those circumstances is likely to disappoint.

Cultures for fungal growth are carried out with the purpose of identifying the causes of individual infections.

Substances responsible for inhalant allergies are pollens (from trees, grasses and weeds), moulds, dust, mites, feathers and dander. Tests for allergies are available and are carried out by injecting small amounts of the substances into the skin and the tests are evaluated 15 to 30 minutes later.

Biopsies are taken for microscopic examination of the full skin thickness.

Immunopathologic examination is used to identify autoantibodies which may be the cause of disease.

Cytology is the microscopic study of free cells.

Serology is the examination of blood serum for the presence of antibodies and could be used in any skin disease of infectious origin.

Complement fixation tests are used for similar purposes, as is the LE (lupus erythematosus) cell test.

Hair analysis is carried out but unproven in value; nutritional imbalances are sometimes discovered in this way and are of dubious importance.

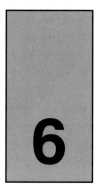

# 6 Wounds

Wounds may be divided into the following categories, always remembering that infinite variations occur in the field and no two wounds are ever the same:

—Abrasions, where only the surface of the skin is damaged and sensitive areas are exposed. These may result from falls on hard surfaces, scraping legs while being loaded onto a trailer or from minor overreaches and brushing.

—Simple skin wounds, caused by sharp instruments in which the wound is clean and free from contamination.

—Contusions, occurring from the effects of falls, kicks, and so on. There is breaking of the skin without parting of the edges.

—Lacerations, with damage to deeper tissues. The edges of the wound are irregular and there is usually an amount of dead tissue.

—Puncture wounds.

—Wounds that involve skin loss.

## Skin Repair

In a simple incision made by a surgeon's knife there is a deliberate attempt to avoid infection and keep the wound clean. The knife will be sterile, the skin treated with bactericidal solutions. Therefore, under ideal circumstances, the wound will heal without infection. The process through which this happens is described below.

Bleeding occurs into the incision and the blood clots. As the clot shrinks the sides of the wound are drawn together and held there by the glue-like properties of the coagulum. White blood cells invade and gradually digest

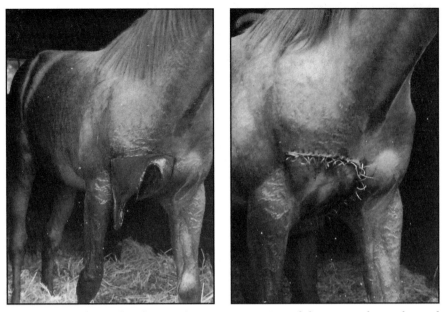

*Laceration* (left) *of the chest with extensive tearing of the pectoral muscle; and* (right) *the same animal after suturing*

the clot; they also remove foreign matter, including bacteria and any dead tissue. Connective tissue cells multiply and small blood vessels invade the area. The purpose of this is to strengthen the repair and provide a new circulation to replace damaged vessels. Surface cells proliferate and close the incision. The process will take about one week to ten days to complete.

There is no discharge from such a wound unless irritants are applied mistakenly to clean it. However, if organisms are introduced, the area becomes inflamed and there will be discharges and local tissue swelling. If the wound has been stitched the reaction will be greater because of inadequate drainage. The stitches may well break down.

## Infected Wound Repair

Infected wounds heal by granulation, the most common form of healing we see. It is based on a combination of fibrous tissue and blood vessel invasion of the damaged area. White cells come in and attack foreign matter in the wound. Once this is completed and the wound if fully filled

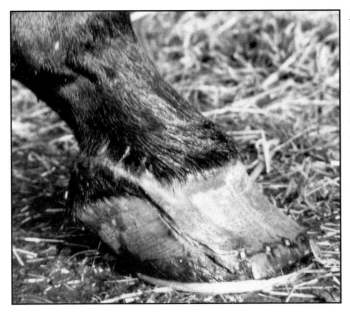

*A coronary injury after repair. The healed wound on the coronet shows the suture line and ensuing defective hoof growth*

by new tissue the wound becomes impervious to further infection. Surface cells will then grow and cover the new tissue which gradually retreats as the healing process completes.

## Other Complications

Where there is excessive movement in a wound (for example, a transverse wound on the front of the knee, or where the two ends of the wound

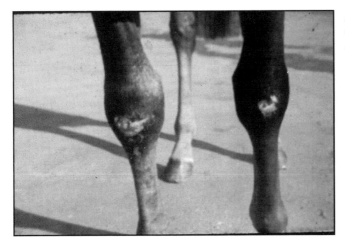

*Broken knees, caused by a fall on the road*

are being dragged apart by gravity influences), there is delayed healing and very often proud flesh. The influence here is exacerbated if the distal skin area has been cut off from its blood supply. In some cases there will be a risk of this skin dying off, an event that may require surgical removal and can complicate repair of the original wound.

## Treatment of Wounds

Because of the variety of wounds seen it is not easy to generalise on treatment. However some basic principles apply.

**Prevent Tetanus**

In the case of all wounds the danger of infection exists. Tetanus, caused by the bacterium, *Clostridium tetani*, is an obvious danger and all horses with surface wounds should have immediate cover, either through the use of antiserum or by annual vaccination, both of which are very effective.

Wounds in which there is the greatest risk of tetanus are puncture wounds or other wounds where there is a possibility of anaerobic conditions developing under the skin.

**Apply First-aid**

First-aid principles demand the control of bleeding and the support of damaged tissues. These may be effected by applying pressure to exposed bleeding points and bandaging the area until treatment can proceed.

A decision on whether or not to suture the wound will be made in the light of several factors such as size, position on the body, degree of contamination, if a section of skin has been lost, ability to cover exposed areas, likely suture tension and so on. These are decisions which will be made by the veterinary surgeon and there are many cases where a wound will heal better without being stitched, but the main consideration is whether the repair process will benefit from the procedure and whether or not it might endanger the animal by not stitching (as with an abdominal wound).

There are some wounds in which severe tissue damage or skin loss will mitigate against the idea of suturing, yet the act of closing off the wound and reducing the size of an exposed area will be beneficial in the long term.

Even though the repair may break down, the process is facilitated by suturing and the final outcome may justify the procedure where large areas of flesh are exposed. However, it is vital that the area be meticulously cleaned and aftercare of the wound is a daily task until repair is completed.

## Clean the Wound

All gross and minute dirt must be picked out. If this is only possible under local anaesthetic, it then becomes a job for the veterinary surgeon. Only very mild, warm solutions should be used for cleaning as more irritant antiseptics will further damage exposed tissues and complicate healing. Boiling water will do the same. No antiseptics or disinfectants should be used unless greatly diluted.

The same procedure will apply to wounds which are being sutured. Thorough cleaning is necessary as any minute dirt left behind can act as a focus of infection which will cause the repair to break down. In fact the first duty of the vet is to remove all vestiges of foreign matter or debilitated tissue.

## Cover the Wound

If the wound is clean and is not being stitched, it may be advisable to cover it if possible. This is done for two reasons: first to limit effusion; second to support the damaged structures and help them to stay in apposition as they knit.

A dressing of wound powder should be applied followed by some sterile cotton wool or gauze. An outer layer of adhesive bandage helps to hold the dressing in place.

A point comes after the initial body reaction has been stemmed when the wound will benefit from exposure to air; and, the earlier this can be achieved without endangering progress, the better for the animal. At this stage a wound powder may be applied to help drying and keep the surface from invasion by bacteria. Prevention of fly contamination should also be considered.

## Apply Dressings

In badly infected wounds it may be necessary to apply poultices, and use injections of antibiotics to control the problem. Gauze dressings impregnated with antibiotic are also helpful applied directly over the wound. To an extent, strong supporting dressings will, through the application of pressure, limit proud flesh.

It may be necessary to replace dressings every twelve or twenty-four hours. On removing the dressing a yellow sticky mass may be seen. This should be gently cleaned away with swabs of cotton wool, using warm saline solution or well diluted antiseptics. The point of the exercise is to help the body by getting rid of the discharges; but do not be too vigorous as it is possible to damage the repairing tissues.

## Physiotherapy

Use of physiotherapy includes treatment by laser and ultrasound therapy. In certain conditions, where there are signs of proud flesh formation, for example, physiotherapy is very effective in promoting good union and stemming excessive growth.

## Open Wounds

Wounds and abrasions which are left open from the start may be treated locally with a suitable wound powder or spray. The main purpose of these will be to kill surface organisms and thus foster healing.

## Dead Tissue

If there is dead tissue this may need to be removed. Flaps of skin which have been cut away from their blood supply are unable to survive and will shrivel up. They may impede repair. A veterinary surgeon will decide; however, in very obvious cases they can be cut off with a blade or scissors.

## Limit Movement

Where the edges of a wound are being pulled apart by natural dynamic factors (as in all transverse limb wounds) it is vital to limit movement. This may be effected by applying bandages which support the tissues and keep the ends together. Alternatively, something stronger like a cast or a splint may have the same effect, although the total exclusion of drainage and air is not beneficial, particularly in infected wounds. This may be overcome to an extent by the use of a window in the cast, allowing the movement to be prevented and the wound cleaned.

## Puncture Wounds

Treatment of puncture wounds requires protection against tetanus and the use of antibiotics, both locally and by injection. It is important also to draw infected material to the surface with poultices. If this is not achieved there is a danger of abscess formation.

## Foreign Bodies

Where foreign bodies such as thorns, for example, have penetrated deeply into tissues, unless they can be seen and withdrawn, there will be a constant chronic reaction which will not heal. Continuous poulticing may draw the wound, or it may be possible to lance the tissues and force the thorn out. Pieces of glass may remain in tissues for years.

### Encourage Drainage
Always encourage drainage and if bathing is necessary – particularly where infection has moved away from the wound – bathe towards the open edges.

If gas is being sucked into a wound and spreading, this should be massaged back towards the opening. This often occurs in areas such as the armpit and the inguinal area, where any movement causes air to be sucked under the skin. Usually this does not complicate repair although the spread of gas may allow the spread of subcutaneous infection. In time this process can be limited through use of ultrasound as long as all infection has been overcome.

### Limit Infection
Where exudate is passively travelling under the skin, with gravity, it is important to limit infection, perhaps with antibiotics, especially as this type of fluid forms an ideal medium for bacterial growth. Occasionally added drainage points have to be created surgically to allow infected matter to escape.

### Exercise
Exercise is important from the time a wound is strong enough to withstand it. This may be confined to a short walk about the box or yard. It helps to strengthen the repair and leave a wound which will not break down when the animal is returned to work.

### Leg Wounds
Virtually all leg wounds cause damage to circulation. This will result in filling of the leg until the situation returns to normality. Where a major vein has been seriously damaged, collateral circulation has to be established. This is sometimes evident on the neck when a jugular vein has been obliterated. A mesh of small veins may appear in the area, which take over the drainage of local tissues. Such an event in a leg would take a considerable time to mend. Controlled exercise is important to hasten the process.

### Establish Damage
Where a wound overlies bone it is important to ensure, by radiography

perhaps, that the bone itself is not damaged. Similarly, by local inspection, the extent of soft tissue damage to, for example, ligaments is established.

**Loss of Skin**
Where there is an almost total loss of skin the animal's ability to survive will depend on the extent of the loss. In some cases an early decision will have to be made on humane destruction. However, where the area is of a manageable size, the important thing is to stem the outflow of serous fluid, to protect the area from contamination, and encourage the edges of skin to close over by degrees. It is remarkable how many big wounds heal successfully and leave quite tidy scarring.

# Proud Flesh

A common consequence of repair in lower limb wounds, proud flesh is identified as an exuberant growth of soft tissue on the surface of the wound, which is usually red, or pink, in colour and moist in texture. It tends to grow rapidly, often becoming as large an an orange, or bigger, and its presence prevents the edges of the wound from coming together.

Proud flesh occurs when there is excessive granulation in wound repair. This appears quite commonly in equine wounds and is more likely in areas where there is skin loss or where mechanical forces result in gaping wounds.

## Clinical Signs

Any wound that repairs without primary healing will usually show exposed areas of granulation which are quite normal. The influence of the granulating process is to draw the skin together by providing a medium over which the repairing cells can grow. However, when granulation tissue produces excessive growth, this appears like a tumour above the skin. It is usually red, or pink, and moist with yellow or grey discharge on its surface.

Affected animals do not like the lesions being touched and they bleed quite easily. Proud flesh may develop uninhibited and grow to the size of a grapefruit or larger.

## Treatment

Where the proud flesh is very large, it may be necessary to remove it surgically. However, it will regrow unless efforts are made to prevent it. The simplest way to achieve this is with instruments like therapeutic ultrasound or lasers which stimulate normal wound repair and inhibit the further development of granulation. In the past, various surface applications have been used, from tissue destructive agents like copper sulphate to preparations containing enzymes like trypsin that digest proud flesh, and many others. Their success varied although enzyme containing sprays were very effective if used with care. However, today, the judicious use of repair-stimulating physiotherapy has eliminated the need for any of these.

# Burns

The occurrence of burns is due to a variety of causes, some of which are discussed here. Such damage can be caused by extreme heat, as in fire or contact with boiling liquids, by extreme cold, as in frostbite or from the effect of acids and alkalis – burns may also be a consequence of exposure to radiation.

Burns are classified according to the degree of skin injury and to the depth of tissue damage they cause. Thus, first-degree burns are classified as superficial and are repaired from the deeper layers of the epidermis. Second-degree burns involve almost the full thickness of the skin. Third-degree burns involve subcutaneous tissues as well as the full skin.

First-degree burns will result in erythroderma, or reddening of the skin, which may go unnoticed on the skin of pigmented animals. In second-degree burns there is exudation from the skin with crust formation and acute local tissue reaction. Third-degree burns cause loss of whole areas of skin which are ultimately replaced by a marked scar.

Where there is fire and animals are subject to the inhalation of toxic fumes, the damage to the respiratory lining tissues may be more significant than damage to skin. In these cases, local tissue reactions could cause death by suffocation. Systemic shock can also result from the effects of severe tissue damage and this too can lead to death.

Secondary bacterial infections may follow local tissue damage and the aftercare of burns must take this into account as a routine.

## Treatment

Consideration must be given to the local and systemic effects of burns. Drugs to control pain may be necessary and treatment for shock may need to be instigated at an early stage. Anti-inflammatory drugs may also be required to control the extent of the tissue reactions. Broad spectrum antibiotics are necessary where there is risk of infection.

Local burn therapy includes the application of moist dressings which help to exclude air. Impregnated gauze sections are useful for this.

If acids or alkalies are the cause of the burn the offending chemical must be washed clean from the affected area and neutralised where this is possible.

Despite the increasing use of electric fencing, horses are not often presented with electric burns. This is more likely to occur where they are in contact with power lines, in which case they are unlikely to survive. Animals affected by lightning are usually found dead and the diagnosis is made post-mortem. In either case, animals that do survive tend to be severely affected and suffer shock and other acute systemic symptoms.

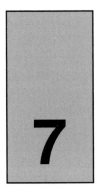

# 7 External Parasites

Ectoparasites live on the surface of the body, or its appendages (like the ear). They include those that live full time on or within the skin (lice, mites, and so on) as well as those that cause their irritation through periodic visits to the host (for example, biting flies).

The effects of skin parasitism usually depend on the size of the invading population, on the manner in which the parasite ekes its existence and on the state of nutrition of the host animal when infected. The damage ectoparasites inflict may be mechanical, but the situation is complicated also by host reactions to the presence of particular parasites, their secretions and excreta.

There is an inevitable difference here between parasites that spend the whole (or most of) their lives on the host, for example, lice and mites, and those, like the various flies, ticks, fleas and so on, that only visit periodically and for varying lengths of time.

High numbers of permanent ectoparasites, in some cases, may be the result of ill-health, not the cause of it. However, the influence of infestation can affect production (for example, it is proven that milk production in cattle and wool growth in sheep suffer). Anaemia has been recognised in lice infestations of horses and is due to blood sucking on the part of the lice.

Heavy infestations of lice on broodmares might also affect milk production, or, as affected mares are often in very poor condition, influence the development of the foal. Of course, these are unproven suggestions, but the implication is there and the very possibility increases the importance of control in such situations.

Diseases caused by ectoparasites, especially flies, are numerous, so horses benefit from the elimination of skin infestations.

*Factors affecting*
*disease resistance*

> • Natural decline with age
> • Malnutrition
> • Intercurrent disease
> • Climatic conditions
> • Exposure
> • Stress

For the purposes of classification ectoparasites are divided into insects and arachnids, the general distinction between them being that insects (the class *Insecta*) have three body segments, three pairs of legs, wings and antennae; arachnids (the class *Arachnida*) have two body segments, four pairs of legs in the adult and no wings or no antennae.

In this chapter we discuss insects and arachnids and we also consider those insects with intermediate stages within a host, like bots and warbles, as well as those that invade skin lesions or cause dermatitis.

We begin with the insects which consist of flies, mosquitoes, lice and fleas. Their distinguishing features are: the possession of wings, three pairs of legs, a head, a thorax and an abdomen. The head contains two eyes, two antennae and a complex set of mouthparts. The thorax consists of three parts and bears six jointed legs. Most have wings (one or two pairs) but some are wingless: roaches (*Dictyophora*), beetles (*Coleoptera*) and certain bugs (*Hemiptera*) have two pairs of wings; most flies (*Diptera*) have one pair, and lice (*Mallophaga* and *Anoplura*) and fleas (*Siphonaptera*) are wingless. The functional wings of *Diptera* arise from the thorax. The abdomen consists of 11 or fewer segments of which the terminal ones are modified for copulation or egg laying.

## Fly Worry

Flies are classified *Diptera* because of the possession of only one pair of wings. Most flies are oviparous (lay eggs), though a few deposit larvae that have already been hatched. There are three main groups: the gnats and mosquitoes of the *Nematocera*, the horse and deerflies of the *Brachycera* and the more highly evolved flies of the *Cyclorrhapha*. All three contain blood–sucking species. They have their effect on a host in several ways:

1. Many species produce localised lesions by the physical act of biting. This may be complicated by the deposition of substances (like saliva and other excretions) which are toxic or capable of causing allergies.
2. By sheer annoyance flies may worry horses to the extent that they stop

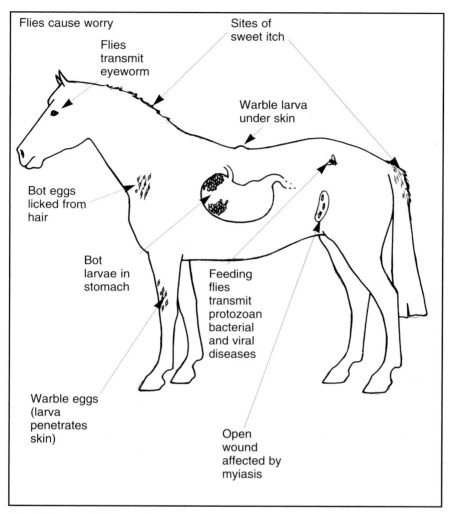

Flies cause worry

Flies transmit eyeworm

Sites of sweet itch

Warble larva under skin

Bot eggs licked from hair

Bot larvae in stomach

Feeding flies transmit protozoan bacterial and viral diseases

Warble eggs (larva penetrates skin)

Open wound affected by myiasis

*The influence of flies on horses*

grazing and lose weight in extreme cases. There may also be incitement to self-trauma as a result of irritation.

3. As vectors of disease: viral, bacterial and parasitic diseases may be spread by flies that become contaminated with discharges and carry these on to unaffected animals, mechanically. It can be appreciated from this that in diseases like equine influenza flies can be significant, especially within relatively tight confines. Viral, and other, diseases are also transmitted by direct injection into the bloodstream by biting flies

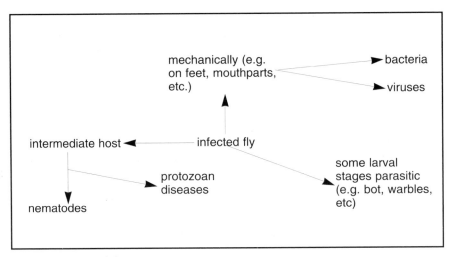

*Flies as agents of disease*

as they feed. Flies also attack wounds and act as carriers of organisms which may set up infection in these situations; castration wounds being a case in point. The intermediate stages of some parasitic diseases are also transmitted, using certain flies as intermediate hosts.

4. Larvae of some flies invade living tissue to cause a condition called myiasis. This includes surface invasion of wounds as well as internal infection by warble and bot flies. As it is the larvae that are parasitic, adults merely serve to deposit eggs on a suitable host. *Dermatobia hominis* (whose larvae are parasites of man, mammals and birds) attaches its eggs to mosquitoes and other host-seeking, biting flies which therefore serve to spread the disease. *Rhinoestrus purpureus* is the head maggot-fly, whose larvae crawl into and develop in the nasal sinuses. This condition is mainly found in remote parts of Europe, Africa and Asia. The *Calliphoridae* include genera such as *Calliphora*, *Lucilia* and *Chrysomya*. Myiasis caused by these parasites occurs only rarely in horses, but *Chrysomya bezziana* and *Cochliomyia hominivorax* do invade and are respectively the screw-worms of the Old and New World.

5. Flies that suck blood do so in order to obtain a source of protein before they begin to lay their eggs. The males of many species are therefore innocuous, feeding mainly on plant juices and not interfering with animals; females alone feeding on blood. The result may be bleeding puncture-wounds or abrasions which can become infected, or weals,

papules and oedematous swellings. The pain they cause may result in anything from head-shaking or tail-switching to intense irritation and restlessness. Most flies only visit the host for a brief spell, but *Haematobia irritans* tends to remain between meals, though capable of flying off.

The flies described below all affect horses as detailed. The control of flies is a matter of understanding their habitats and life cycles, the use of insecticides, where available, and protecting animals such as horses from attack through good stable hygiene, or by the use of screens and nets where there is a particular problem.

## Midges (*Culicoides*)

Midges, *Culicoides* species, are minute flies (some 0.5mm to 3mm long) belonging to the nematoceran family *Ceratopogonidae*, which have specially adapted mouth parts for biting and sucking blood. They are a widespread nuisance and the cause of sweet itch in the horse.

*C. pulicaris* is the species thought to be most commonly associated with sweet itch in the UK and Ireland. Over 800 species are known, each with its own feeding preferences, ranging from stealing blood from engorged mosquitoes to biting specific parts of the body of domestic animals. On horses, *C. pulicaris* feeds mostly on the mane and tail (areas of coarsest hair) and *C. nubeculosus* goes for the underside of the body.

Sweet itch is seasonal and recurring and appears in individual animals (about 3 per cent of British ponies) during the warmer months, from April/May to November, when the flies are about. There is a suggestion that predisposition to sweet itch is hereditary, although some animals seem to recover fully. While it may well be that there is an hereditary basis, this is not the only cause, nor does the idea provide a simple answer to the problem. However, it might be wise to avoid breeding from those animals suffering particularly intractable cases of the disease.

## Life Cycle

*Culicoides* larvae are all aquatic or semi-aquatic. The eggs are laid in water and the worm-like larvae are found in mud, around lakes, ponds and rivers. After undergoing a pupal stage, the adult fly emerges and these attack the horse (usually not straying more than a few hundred

*Adult* Culicoides, *cause of sweet itch*

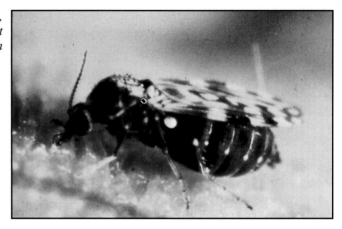

metres from their breeding area in doing so), causing a reaction that is at least partly an allergic dermatitis. The saliva of a few species, for example, *C. pulicaris* in the UK and Ireland and *C. robertsi* in Australia appears to contain a factor that initiates an intense allergic response.

Sweet itch, which is also sometimes known as 'summer dermatitis' or 'Queensland itch', depending on geographical location, is widespread and particular animals seem to be more susceptible than others. *Culicoides* flies may appear in swarms. *C. pulicaris* breeds in swampy areas, *C. nebeculosus* uses wet soil fouled with faecal material.

Population numbers of midges are influenced by climatic factors. For example, *C. pulicaris* shows peaks of activity in May and September in southern England, whereas in Scotland it is June and July.

Only the females bite, but they cause great annoyance. Some species of *Culicoides* act as vectors for serious viral diseases such as African horse sickness and Venezuelan equine encephalitis, while *C. nubeculosis* acts as an intermediate host for the filarial nematode *Onchocerca cervicalis*.

## Identifying Features

A significant factor is the extremely small size of these flies. In finer detail, the antennae are long and slender and the proboscis (mouthpart) is short.

## Clinical Signs

Sweet itch is not difficult to recognise. Lesions are seasonal and observed mainly on the crest and tail of the horse. The lesions can begin as small papules which lead to considerable raw areas as a result of itching.

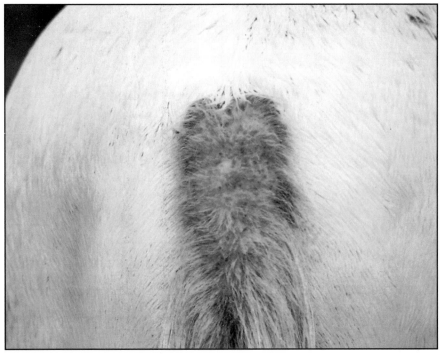

*A typical sweet itch lesion* (above) *on the tail of a Welsh pony; and (*below*), in the shoulder region, the same pony showing fly-bite reactions*

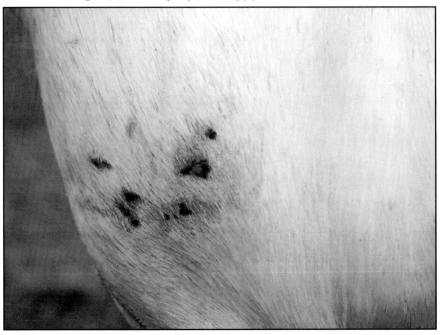

Affected horses suffer severe pruritis which may lead to self-inflicted injuries from scratching against sharp objects.

The condition usually appears first when horses are aged between one and five years. Only small numbers within groups are affected and symptoms are more likely to be seen in animals at grass than in those kept indoors.

## Diagnosis

Although recognition of sweet itch presents no difficulty, there are varying degrees of susceptibility – some animals may suffer the condition for a period, or for a season and not show signs again. The occurrence is related to the fly season, and the predominance of neck and tail lesions with acute itching is typical.

Irritation of the ventral abdomen due to *C. nubeculosus* may be confused with symptoms caused by other flies or by contact dermatitis. Tail scratching can be caused by pinworms, and similar problems with the mane may result from such diverse causes as selenium toxicity, mange or ringworm.

## Control

Stabling horses helps control the incidence of sweet itch during periods while the fly is on the wing. Flies are most active on mild, humid still days, particularly at daybreak and nightfall. In some areas this means stabling affected animals before 4.00 p.m. until 10.00 a.m.

There is no doubt that sweet itch can be a considerable problem in individual animals and be very difficult to deal with. Keeping affected horses out of marshy fields and away from rivers and lakes is helpful, especially if they do not have ready access to surfaces on which to scratch (such as trees and posts). Fly screens are used on stable doors, windows and other inlets; however, the fly is so small it may penetrate even very fine meshes.

The only logical approach to prevention at present is to protect the animal from contact with the causative fly.

However, in spite of these precautions, the condition may still occur and the treatment of lesions with drugs to reduce inflammation and soothe already exposed areas is often necessary.

## Treatment

Insecticides are used on individual animals with varying degrees of success, either applied locally or as impregnated tags attached to headcollars and the like. Particularly susceptible animals make topical preventive treatments appear disappointing. Antihistamines may aid regression of the lesions and long-acting corticosteroids are used by some veterinarians as a routine treatment; however, the possible side effects have to be understood as this drug is an anti-inflammatory and may influence body reactions to other encountered infections.

The prospect for the future is the hope that immunotherapy may allow for the production of an antigen against *Culicoides* and that animals may be capable of being successfully protected in this way.

---

- The first priority is to prevent fly bites
- Stable animals at critical times
- Use fly deterrents, screens, protective gear
- Avoid marshy fields, rivers, lakes
- Avoid trees, posts (for scratching), etc., wherever possible
- Insecticides, applied regularly, help to keep flies at bay
- Modern horse clothing covers the whole body, with holes for the eyes and ears; or, sections (e.g. for head, neck and mane) may only be covered
- Fly fringes and tags also contain insecticides and may help in keeping flies at bay

*Summary chart: sweet itch*

## Stable Fly (*Stomoxys*)

The stable fly, *Stomoxys calcitrans*, sucks blood and also may cause an allergic reaction. It is much the same size as the common house fly, its bite is very painful and irritating and the wounds inflicted by it may bleed freely afterwards.

World-wide in distribution, the stable fly is important as a transmitter of diseases such as equine infectious anaemia (EIA), some trypanosomes, *Habronema* and *Setaria* species, also *Dermatophilus congolensis*, the cause of rain scald and mud fever (mycotic dermatitis). Its saliva may also cause allergic reactions.

Females lay their eggs in decaying matter, sometimes horse manure. As many as 800 eggs may be laid about one week after maturation; from these larvae hatch in some two to four days. The larvae mature to adults in 14 to 24 days. Before egg laying, females must first feed from a horse or other animal, or even man.

Stable fly bites are seen on the skin as small red bumps that may be still bleeding when fresh. If present in large numbers they may cause skin crusting and hair loss. In control, it is important to remove any material from stables that may act as a breeding ground for this fly. Muck heaps should be remote from the stable yard. Insecticides may have an effect on areas (like sunny walls) where the flies rest.

Local lesions may have to be treated when severe with drugs of an anti-inflammatory type and insect repellants used to keep flies at bay.

## House Fly (*Musca*)

The house fly, *Musca domestica*, is attracted to wounds and to the moist parts of the body, like the eyes, where it can provoke dermatitis. It is also attracted to discharges, like those from the mare's uterus, and helps to irritate local tissues by its presence.

*Musca* can act as a mechnical vector of *Habronema* and *Thelazia* species. It also transports *Draschia megastoma* and *Habronema muscae* (cultaneous Habronomiasis), the nematode parasites of the horse's stomach. Many closely related species of fly act in the same way. *Musca* can use alternative sources of food, from faeces to decomposing fruit, from natural secretions to almost any soluble material. Eggs are laid in clusters in decaying organic matter and hatch within hours. The larvae of *Musca* species are typical 'maggots'. After two moults a pupa is formed from which an adult emerges in two to three weeks. *Musca* species adults mechanically carry disease organisms on their feet and body hairs, also through their feeding habits and own excretions.

Another member of this family affecting horses is *Musca autumnalis*, the face fly, which is also implicated in the transmission of pinkeye in cattle.

*Haematobia irritans*, the horn fly of cattle, is another biting muscid. It is similar to, but smaller than, the stable fly. It transmits diseases such as surra, cutaneous habronemiasis and eye-worm.

*Hydrotoea irritans*, another biting muscid, acts in a similar way but is more irritating to the horse by scratching the skin and provoking the release of blood and tissue fluids.

## Horse Fly (*Tabanus*)

The horse fly, *Tabanus*, is a large fly with colourless wings that lays its eggs on vegetation over water or wet soil. Females require a blood meal for egg development but also use other sources of food, such as nectar and sap. Larvae hatch in about one week and usually drop into water. Third-stage larvae of aquatic species are voracious carnivores and live on other insect larvae, snails, earthworms and dead organic matter. Some larvae have the capacity to over-winter in moderate climates.

*Chrysops* (the deer fly) and *Haematopota* are closely related to the horse fly. Horses fear these flies because of the deep bites they inflict when females feed.

Horse flies are effective disease transmitters, for example, EIA and trypanosomiasis.

*Simulium* species are smaller and very similar to horse flies; they are also biting flies which may cause weals to form, especially within the ear. They tend to occur in swarms and have been known to cause death of animals, probably from worry. Some species transmit the virus of equine viral encephalomyelitis.

Simulids are world-wide in distribution. They lay their eggs on aquatic vegetation in swift-flowing water but may travel as far as 15km from their breeding grounds to feed. The larvae are tiny, black and spindle-shaped.

## Tsetse Fly (*Glossina*)

The tsetse fly, *Glossina sp.*, found in Africa south of the Sahara, is a wasp-like fly, which is an obligatory blood feeder. It transmits the protozoan disease, trypanosomiasis.

## Hippoboscids (*Hippobosca*)

The adult hippoboscids are blood-sucking flies found mainly in the UK and are adapted for a permanent ectoparasitic existence. These include the forest fly, *Hippobosca equina*, found mostly under the tail and between the hind legs of horses. Hippoboscids and tsetse flies retain their larvae within their abdomens and these pupate almost immediately on being born.

## Mosquitoes

Over 3,000 species of mosquito exist, many belonging to the genera *Culex*, *Aedes* and *Anopheles*. They transmit the Venezuelan and eastern encephalitis viruses and the filarial parasite *Setaria*.

Mosquito females feed directly from blood vessels, through a slender tube that extends from the mouth. The male feeds on plant juices and is distinguished from the female by the shape of its antennae. All juvenile forms are aquatic. Larvae have a breathing siphon and hang from the water surface. The mosquito causes irritation by biting and varying degrees of skin reaction occur. Most mosquitoes bite at night, therefore suitable netting may protect animals housed at this time.

Treatment is with pyrethrum or other available insecticides.

## Blowfly, Screw-worm

The blowfly and the screw-worm are both to be found in horses in tropical countries and occur when flies lay their eggs in and around the edges of wounds. The eggs develop into larvae (maggots) about 1.5cm in size.

*Blowfly larvae, a cause of myiasis*

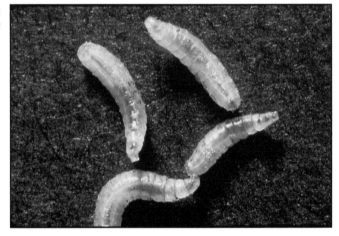

*Adult* Lucilia, *the blowfly*

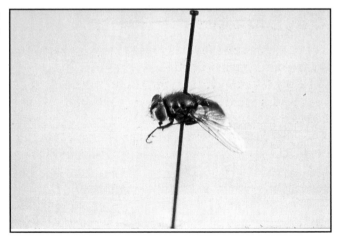

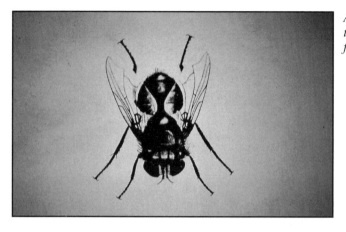

*Adult* Chrysomia, *the screw-worm fly*

The larvae feed on dead matter within the wound and may add to the tissue damage by releasing toxins that affect surrounding tissues. After this stage of their development, the larvae drop to the ground where they pupate and become flies.

The infection of a wound with larvae is called myiasis. Treatment of the problem involves removal of the larvae, cleansing of the wound and the stimulation of normal tissue repair.

Blowflies belong to the *Lucilia* family. Screw-worms belong to the *Chrysomia* and *Cochliomyia* families.

Screw-worm adult flies lay eggs at the edges of new wounds and body openings. Eggs hatch in 10 to 12 hours and the larvae mature in the wounds in three to six days. The lesions are severe and cause necrosis with smell from the wounds.

## Wasps and Bees

The wasp, *Polestes humitis*, belongs to the order *Hymenoptera* and causes local irritation where it stings.

Bees can cause acute local reactions to their sting and are capable of causing a systemic effect in horses which can include diarrhoea, blood-containing urine, jaundice and collapse. This is caused by the honey bee, *Apis mellifera*.

## Botfly

Botflies are not a major cause of skin disease in horses but are included here because of their close relationship to other flies under discussion. The adult flies contribute to the effect of fly worry, but the major disease influence of bots is as endoparasites in the mouth and stomach.

The horse botfly is *Gasterophilus intestinalis*; other associated species include *G. nasalis* (throat botfly) and *G. haemorrhoidalis* (nose botfly). *G. intestinalis* and *G. nasalis* are worldwide in distribution, while *G. haemmorhoidalis* is not so common. Research has shown that 90 per cent of horses have been found infected with bots.

The clinical importance of bots is often disputed as it is the larval stages which are parasitic and these enter the host and eventually inhabit the stomach where they over-winter. Bots may be found in large numbers at this time, though the destruction they cause is not considered great. They may also be found in the pharynx, duodenum and rectum. Bots attach to the stomach lining and are often present in sufficient numbers to influence digestion, perhaps even blocking the entrance to the stomach from the oesophagus. The site of their attachment is marked by a deep ulcer around which the tissue is thickened. They may cause haemorrhage and occasional bots may burrow through the wall of the stomach and cause peritonitis, but this is extremely rare. In addition, adult botflies cause considerable worry to horses, who tend to resent their approach and show signs of apprehension; others may gallop to avoid egg-laying females, who deposit their eggs on the limb and body hairs.

After gaining entry to a host, the migration of larvae through the tissues of the mouth and cheeks may cause considerable discomfort and could cause loss of condition in animals suffering heavy infestations.

Bot larvae spend about ten months inside the host; they spend two months externally in which they complete pupation, find a new host, and lay eggs which develop to an infective stage. Actually the eggs hatch in response to the warmth produced by a horse's muzzle and breath and then enter the mouth, usually when licked off the hair.

## Life Cycle

The adult fly lays its eggs singly on the hairs of the host animal in the summer months. These eggs are yellow, clearly visible and are often distributed in patches or rows which are difficult to remove by hand or brush. Each female may lay as many as 1,000 eggs.

The eggs of *G. intestinalis* hatch under the influence of moisture, perhaps encouraged by licking, and this takes about seven days to occur. *G. nasalis*, on the other hand, lays about 500 eggs around the chin and throat and these hatch in about one week, unaided.

*G. haemorrhoidalis* lays about 150 black coloured eggs which are deposited about the lips and mouth and may hatch in two to three days. *G. intestinalis* larvae are about 1mm long when entering the host. They remain in the mouth for about three weeks, burrowing through the soft tissues until they emerge and moult, being now some 6mm to 7mm long, and pass on to the stomach after a short period of attachment to the base of the tongue. *G. nasalis* and *G. haemorrhoidalis* both burrow through the skin to gain entry to the host's mouth from where they invade the soft tissues of the tongue and cheeks. After anything up to a month, the larvae of all three species then migrate to the stomach where they spend the winter months.

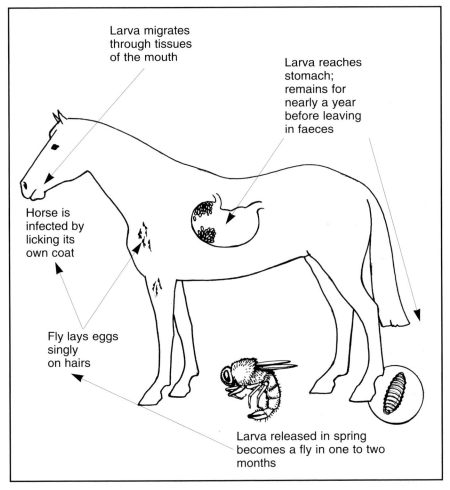

*Life cycle of botfly*

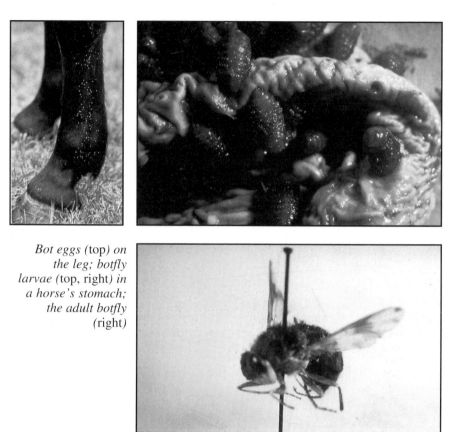

*Bot eggs* (top) *on the leg; botfly larvae* (top, right) *in a horse's stomach; the adult botfly* (right)

On emergence from the horse, larvae leave the dung and enter soil in which they pupate and may take anything from three to ten weeks to develop into an adult fly.

## Identifying Features

The adult fly is a brown, bee-like insect about 18mm long, bearing one pair of wings. The reddish-brown mature larva is approximately 2cm long by 1 cm wide and resides in the stomach of the horse. Its rounded body tapers to a narrow anterior.

## Diagnosis

The eggs on the body, limbs and mane of horses, are easily recognised. They are usually seen as rows of small yellow dots on the hair of the horse's legs and are distinguished from other foreign material by their resistance to brushing. Bot larvae are seen in the droppings as they emerge in the faeces. They may also appear after dosing with an effective drug.

## Control and Treatment

It is an important part of horse management to remove bot eggs when these are present in the coat. This may be done using the special knife for the purpose sold by saddlers, or by judicious use of a blade, or by a strong brush. Providing shelter for the horse from flies may also help, but is impractical in some situations. Horses should be treated with an effective drug in the autumn, when the flies have died off and the larvae have reached the stomach. It is usual to wait for a month after the first severe frost before doing this. Ivermectin is effective against the oral and gastric stages and is safer than the old remedy, carbon disulphide. Dichlorvos and trichlorfon have also been used with some success in the past.

---

- Adult flies lay eggs singly on hair in summer
- Infectious larvae develop in five days
- Larvae burrow through tissues of mouth
- Larvae in stomach attach for as long as ten months
- Larvae leave stomach in late spring
- Adult flies develop in three to nine weeks

---

*Summary chart: botfly*

# Warble Fly

The warble fly, *Hypoderma bovis*, is bee-like and hairy, measuring about 1.5cm long. The mature larvae measure anything up to 3cm and are similar in conformation to the botfly.

Warble flies are more commonly parasites of cattle and deer, but their incidence has greatly decreased in modern times with the advent of schemes which have used effective (mainly organophosphorus) drugs to reduce the damage they were causing to cattle hides. Warbles do not appear to be a natural parasite of horses and the larvae usually fail to thrive and rarely mature fully in the horse.

The eggs are similar in shape and colour to the eggs of the botfly, but are insignificant and seldom seen with the naked eye. Adult flies do not bite but deposit the eggs on the limbs and lower bodies of cattle and horses. The flies are greatly resented and 'gadding' (running away from the fly) has been a considered source of economic loss in cattle when the fly was more plentiful. Eggs hatch in two to seven days. The larvae that emerge burrow through the skin into subcutaneous tissues through which they wander for several months. Eventually they appear as sizeable swellings under the skin of the back of the host where they bore breathing holes and remain for as long as three months. Occasional warbles may find their way to the brain, where they can prove fatal.

In early summer larvae emerge through the breathing pore, and fall to the ground where they pupate. Adults emerge from these pupae in five to six weeks, depending on prevailing conditions, and live for about one week in which they continue the cycle.

Larvae developing under the saddle area of ridden horses can be a major problem, though it is not always easy to distinguish between them and painful galls caused by improperly fitting tack.

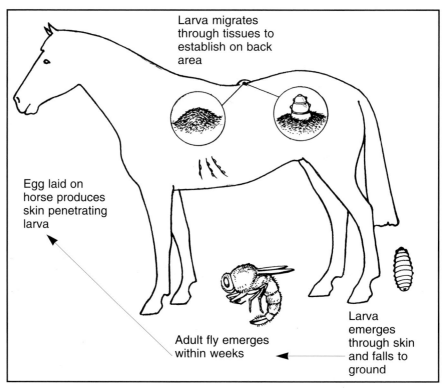

*Life cycle of warble fly*

Local tissue reactions may also occur in response to the presence of the adult larvae, causing acute irritation and serious problems in treatment.

The distinction between warble larvae and painful saddle galls is really only confirmed on the identification of a larva which may be encouraged to emerge from its breathing pore. However, it is not advisable to interfere as it is possible to rupture the warble and set up a severe local tissue reaction.

If the presence of a warble is suspected, the matter must be referred to a veterinary surgeon, as the lesion requires proper diagnosis and treatment. Surgery may be necessary, but the proviso exists that rupture of the warble may lead to an acute local or systemic reaction.

Horses in contact with infested cattle are clearly at risk and may benefit from treatment with insecticide drugs which have proved effective in cattle. Ivermectin is also effective now. But drugs for this problem must be used immediately after the fly season has ended. Adverse reactions occur when larvae are killed during tissue migration; the symptoms being due to toxins released by the dead parasite and the effect may be severe.

---

- Lesions on back are more likely to be saddle galls
- There is a very low incidence of warbles in horses today

---

*Summary chart of warble fly*

# Lice

Lice are small insects with strong claws and no eyes which live as permanent parasites on the skin of warm-blooded animals. They are host-specific, meaning they do not transfer between one type of animal and another. Horse lice passed on to humans may be very irritating for a few hours but no longer than that; they will soon die.

The saliva and faeces of lice contain substances which are capable of causing allergies; giving rise to severe irritation, followed by skin thickening (hyperkeratosis) and, sometimes, self-trauma.

Lice are often present in light infestations which go unnoticed; but the animals acting as host in this case may be the source of infection for others. Large numbers tend to develop on horses that are poor in condition or suffering from other intercurrent diseases, especially in winter when the heavy coat provides an ideal microclimate for louse infestation.

Pediculosis is the name given to infestation with lice.

## Life Cycle

The life cycle of lice lasts about one month, during which time the louse does not leave the host. The eggs can be distinguished from bot and warble-fly eggs by their smaller size and the manner of their attachment to the hair.

There are three nymphal stages in louse development. Transmission is by direct contact, through grooming, or by means of walls, pillars and posts onto which they are passed by scratching animals. Lice do not live long off an animal host. *Haematopinus asini*, a parasite of horses, measures about 3mm in length as an adult and is found in the mane, tail and feather. *Damalinia equi* grows to about 2mm in length. It prefers short-haired areas.

## Identifying Features

Lice have no wings and are flattened from above to below. There are two distinct groups: *Anoplura* (for example, *Hematopinus asini*), which are sucking lice, and *Mallophaga* (for example, *Damalinia equi*), which are chewing lice.

The *Mallophaga* have strong mouths with numerous teeth used for rasping epidermal scales. In the *Anoplura*, mouthparts are much simpler. They attach to the skin by a circlet of teeth and their proboscis is pushed into the deeper tissues. Saliva is pumped into the wound and blood or tissue fluids withdrawn.

## Clinical Signs

Lice are easily seen as very small white specks on the hair and skin. They are distinguished from scurf or dirt by the presence of eggs on the hair and by recognisable movement seen with the naked eye. In heavy infestations there is hair loss and self-trauma from scratching against hard surfaces.

Badly-affected horses may suffer weight loss and become anaemic. However, while younger animals are most severely affected, it is suggested

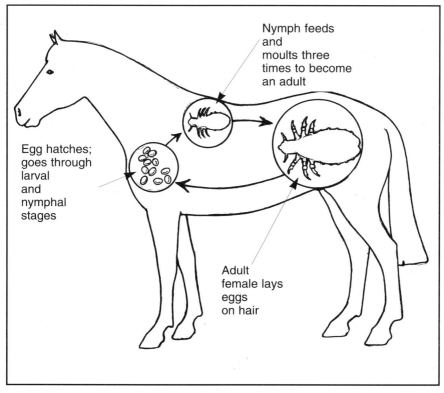

*Life cycle of louse*

that heavy infestations occur in horses whose immunity is already weakened through dietary problems or because of intercurrent disease.

## Diagnosis

Diagnosis is confirmed by identification of the offending louse. The degree of infestation is influenced by diet, and by stresses such as over-crowding, inclement weather, and so on.

## Control and Treatment

Lice are sensitive to a whole range of insecticide sprays or powders, many of which (for example, Lindane) have now been withdrawn from public availability in the UK and Ireland. It should be appreciated that

*Louse infestation causing extensive loss of hair through scratching*

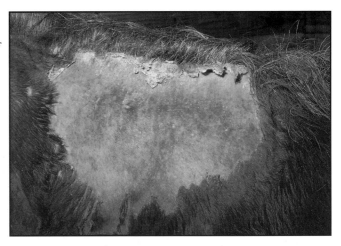

this situation is far from settled at the time of writing (1995) and the prospect is that a wider selection of ectoparasiticides may again be available. However, it must be remembered that treatment should also consider contact animals as well as fixtures and fittings, tack and other possible sources, such as field shelters, scratching posts, and so on. Two spray applications at a two-week interval should suffice with drugs containing coumaphos or pyrethroids (both of which are still available under various proprietary names).

Lice are so susceptible to treatment that elimination is not a major problem under normal circumstances. They are also susceptible to ivermectin and are likely to be eliminated where this drug is used in routine endoparasite control.

An essential part of control where there are heavy infestations is the sterilisation of stables either by pressure hosing or steam-cleaning and the

*A biting louse*

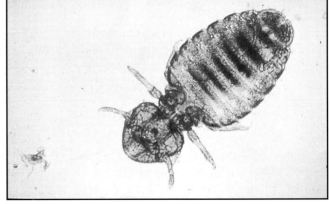

treatment of all wooden surfaces, including fencing posts with creosote or other suitable agent.

# Fleas

Fleas found in the UK and Ireland are not usually associated with infestation of horses. Two varieties of flea found in tropical countries are *Tunga* and *Echidnophaga* and these have been a cause of irritation and skin lesions where they have been found on horses.

Diagnosis is based on the presence of the fleas and treatment must include dusting the local environment with an anti-flea agent (for example, dichlorvos).

Up to this point we have discussed those ectoparasites classified at the beginning of this chapter as *Insecta*. We now turn to those which belong to the class *Arachnida*, with a look at mites, responsible for mange, and ticks.

# Mites

Mites belong to the class *Arachnida* and have four pairs of legs in all except the larval stage. They are responsible for the condition called mange, but there are distinctions in the way individual species cause disease, reflecting anatomy, life style and habitat. Mites are minute in size with piercing mouthparts similar to those of ticks amd most mites are free living; those that live on animals feed on tissue fluids and exudates.

The forage mite, *Tyrophagus*, is a scavanger in stored food but can cause dermatitis when found on animals.

The harvest mite, *Neotrombicula*, is free-living in all but the larval stage which is an obligatory parasite.

Important groups, like *Sarcoptes*, *Psoroptes* and *Chorioptes* dwell permanently on the body surface, while female *Sarcoptes* burrow into the skin to lay their eggs. *Demodex*, which is cigar-shaped, and harmless to horses under normal circumstances, completes its life cycle deep in hair follicles and sebaceous ducts. It may become significant in immune compromised animals. *Notoedres* and *Otodectes* species are also causes of specific types of mange.

While mites that live permanently on their hosts are often host-specific, some can be transmitted to other species, though their ability to exist may be limited on the new host.

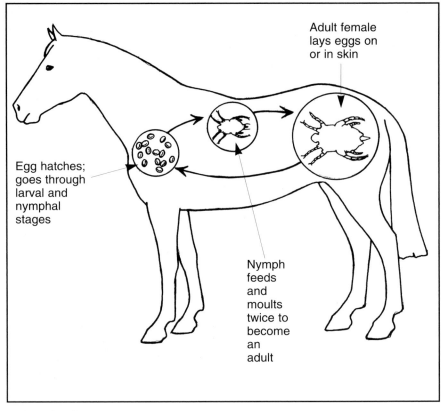

*Life cycle of mite*

Much of the irritation caused by mites is due to hypersensitivity to secretory or excretory products (such as saliva and faeces) and the reaction this creates can lead to self-trauma from scratching.

## Varieties of Mange

Although mange is almost unheard of in horses in the UK and Ireland today, it is still important that the reader be aware of its possibility. There are varieties of mange and some of these are discussed below.

### Sarcoptic Mange

Caused by *Sarcoptes scabei var equi*, sarcoptic mange was until recently a notifiable disease of horses. It induces intense irritation and has been transmitted from horse to man (the condition called 'cavalryman's itch'), but the mites do not establish on the new host and the infection regresses spontaneously. Sarcoptic mange occurs on the face, neck and flank of horses, but is thankfully a rare condition now except in some parts of the Middle East.

The life cycle of the mite takes about two to three weeks to complete, with the females burrowed into the epidermis where they lay their eggs. From each egg a larva hatches which has only six legs. Off the host, mites may persist in the surroundings for several weeks.

The symptoms are related to the irritation and begin with the development of local, small vesicles with hair loss; this may progress to severe scaling with crusting and scarring of the skin as a result of scratching.

Diagnosis is based on symptoms and identification of the causal mite. However, it can be difficult to find the mite on skin scrapings and therefore a negative finding means little in these circumstances. Microscopic examination of skin biopsies shows non-specific inflammation in the absence of actual mites, but the presence of tunnels in the skin and waste products of the mite will suggest a diagnosis.

Various washes, like lime sulphur 5 per cent, lindane (not now available) and so on are effective, though treatment may need to be repeated. The parasite is also susceptible to ivermectin. It is critical to deal with in-contact animals as well as areas in which the parasite is likely to persist off the host.

**Psoroptic Mange**
Caused by *Psoroptes equi*, psoroptic mange (also formerly notifiable) is seen principally on the horse's mane and tail. It is a highly contagious disease the incidence of which is fortunately very low; and the causal mite is host-specific.

This mite does not burrow into the skin like *Sarcoptes* but exists on the surface, feeding off epidermal debris; its life cycle is about the same length and it too can live off the host for two to three weeks.

The degree of irritation is less than with sarcoptic mange, though there is usually plenty of scratching. The head and ears may be affected as well as the mane and tail, resulting in head shaking.

The diagnosis is similarly based on identification of the mite, which is equally as difficult to locate. Treatment follows the same lines but treatment of ear infestation is important where it occurs. Ivermectin has been found effective in this situation.

*Psoroptes cuniculi* lives in the ears and is seen through the otoscope (an instrument for examining the ear) as quickly moving white specks. It

Psoroptes, *equine mange mite*

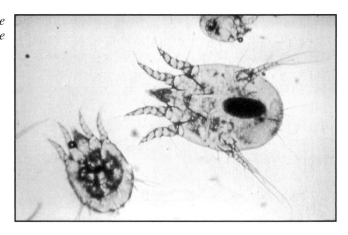

provokes a brown exudate and the irritation can make horses very nervous. Severe cases may cause head-shaking or damage to the base of the ear.

Mange lesions begin as itchy areas covered with small papules. Later the skin becomes thickened and a serous exudate appears which matts the hair and forms crusts. Hair may be lost.

## Chorioptic Mange

*Chorioptes equi*, a host-specific mite, is the cause of chorioptic mange. It affects the legs of heavily-feathered horses and causes irritability and foot

*Lesions of chorioptic mange on the limbs of a horse*

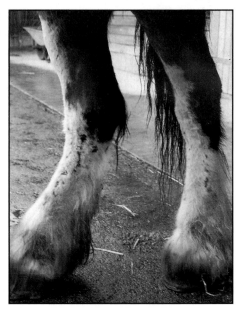

stamping. Though not very contagious direct transmission does occur. The life cycle is about the same length as for both previous mites but *Chorioptes* does not survive off the host for more than a few days. The mite may also parasitise the perineal area.

Diagnosis depends on identification of the mite, which poses the same problems as before and treatment is achieved using the same drugs as for other mite infestations. Ivermectin is effective against this mite.

## Harvest Mite

The larvae of the harvest mite, *Neotrombicula*, are called chiggers and are observed on horses that have encountered wooded areas where the mite parasitises rodents, birds and snakes and other animals. *Neotrombicula* is found in the USA and elsewhere.

Adults are free-living and non-parasitic, but the larvae are obligatory parasites and cause acute irritation to their host on whose skin they remain for several days. They feed by dissolving host cells and using them as food. Lesions usually occur on the head and legs of the host in

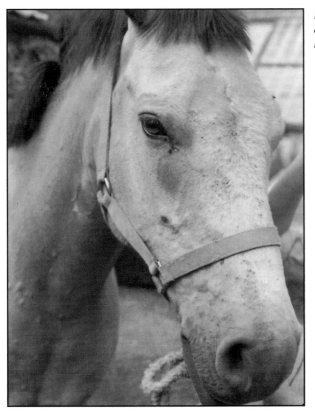

*Horse with infection on face caused by harvest mite*

which the larvae may be seen as small orange dots. The larvae are susceptible to most insecticides but the residual irritation may last for several days after treatment.

**Forage Mite**

A forage mite, *Tyrophagus*, is found in stored products and is capable of causing irritation if finding its way onto horses. The red poultry mite, *Dermanyssus*, requires blood and may also find its way onto horses and is significant in that adults can live free for months off a host.

Forage and harvest mites may feed off horses and may be the cause of heel bug in summer and autumn.

**Demodectic Mange**

*Demodex equi* is a mite which may be a normal inhabitant of equine skin. It exists in the hair follicles and is generally not a cause of irritation in this capacity, acting more the part of a skin commensal than a parasite. The life cycle of *Demodex equi* takes about four to five weeks to complete.

Where there is evident parasitism with this mite, resulting in skin irritation and large areas of hair loss, it is considered that the critical factor is a deficiency of immunity, which may well be genetic in origin in some animals, or could result from the use of corticosteroids.

Diagnosis is relatively easy in these situations as the mites are numerous and found in hair follicles or in the material extruded from them when squeezed. Where the condition has followed corticosteroid therapy, simply withdrawing the drug may result in a cure. However, where the problem persists, treatment with drugs may be considered but this would only be carried out under professional advice because of risks to the horse and precautions to be taken in their use.

Acariasis is the name used when horses are infested with various mites and ticks.

## Ticks

Much larger than mites, ticks are blood-sucking obligatory parasites. They are subdivided into hard (*Ixodidae*) and soft (*Argasidae*) ticks, depending on the presence or absence of a dorsal shield. Only some ticks are host specific (for example, *Dermacentor nitens*, the tropical horse tick); most can feed from a variety of animals. There is a wide range: *Amblyomma*, *Boophilus*, *Dermacentor*, *Ixodes*, *Margaropus*, *Otobius* and *Rhipicephalus*.

Most ticks spend more time off than on the host, but are totally dependent on the host for sustenance. They are subject to micro-environmental factors when on the ground, and thus tend to be endemic in specific types of area. Ticks can exist for very prolonged periods without feeding.

Some ticks are found in wet areas or during a wet season, others can exist in temperate conditions when the appropriate micro-environment exists. The *Argasidae* can survive in a very dry environment.

## Life Cycle

There are three stages: larva, nymph and adult, each of which has to get a blood meal. Soft ticks have several nymphal stages but hard ticks have only one. In some cases, all stages develop on the same animal: one-host ticks. With others, the nymph drops off to moult on the ground so that the new adult has to find a new host. Three-host ticks use a different host for each developmental stage.

The engorged female usually leaves the host to lay her eggs (several thousand) on the ground.

When seeking a new host, ticks climb vegetation to wait. The life cycle extends from as short as three weeks in the tropics to as long as three years in temperate areas.

## Identifying Features

Ticks are recognised on the host as small but usually swollen objects. They are about 1 cm long and firmly attached and increase in size as they feed. They have an unsegmented body and eight legs in all but the larval stage. The shield of the hard tick covers the whole of the small male but only part of the female.

Many species of hard tick bite horses: for example, *Haemaphysalis longicornis* in New Zealand, *Hyalomma anatolicum* in Asia Minor, *Ixodes ricinus* in Europe and *Dermacentor nitens* in Central America.

Soft ticks have no scutum (shield). Both males and females engorge when feeding on a host. They generally feed on birds but *Otobius megnini*, the spinose ear tick, attacks the ears of horses and other animals in the Americas and southern Africa.

## Clinical Signs

Ticks can cause local irritation by attachment, which may lead to secondary infection and ulceration. These wounds attract flies.

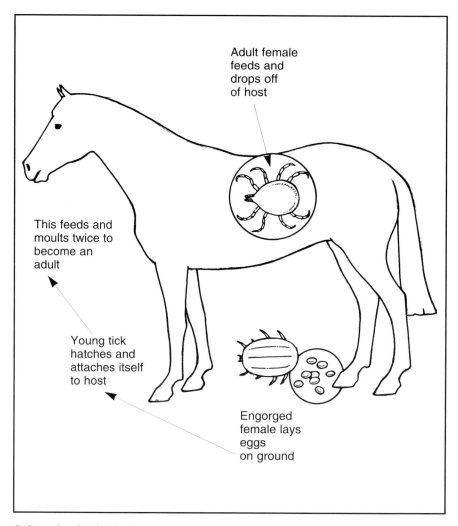

*Life cycle of tick. This process may involve one, two or three hosts, depending on the specific tick*

Each adult female imbibes from 0.5 ml to 2.0 ml of blood while attached to the host, therefore large infestations may lead to anaemia.

The saliva of certain species contains a toxin capable of causing paralysis. In Australia, mature horses as well as foals can succumb to bites from *Ixodes holocyclus*, which usually feeds on the bandicoot.

Ticks may act as vectors for a wide range of diseases, of which equine babesiosis is important. Also transmitted are viral, bacterial, rickettsial and other protozoan diseases.

Tick bites are also capable of causing allergies. There is, therefore, a complex reaction to a tick bite, which is compounded by previous exposure: there is necrosis and lysis of tissues, an influx of inflammatory cells, oedema and hyperplasia of epidermal cells. Fewer ticks will be able to feed on an immune host.

All hard and soft ticks are parasitic, feeding solely on blood and liquified tissues. Their bite is relatively painless, but invasions by large numbers are debilitating. They lacerate tissues and penetrate the epidermis. They tend to feed at varying depths according to species, and some secrete a cementing substance which is why it is so difficult to remove them without leaving the mouthparts behind. Feeding involves pumping saliva into the wound and sucking out dissolved tissue. Hard ticks take

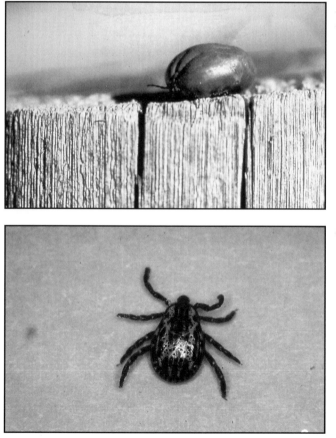

*Engorged female tick*

*Ornate tick*

several days to engorge while soft ticks, with the exception of *Otobius*, feed swiftly and at night.

## Diagnosis

In heavy infestations it is important to identify the causal tick. Unusual varieties are submitted to identification at specialist laboratories.

## Control and Treatment

Control involves avoiding the habitats of the tick. Some tend to inhabit woodland, others rough pasture where they wait on the long grass for a passing host.

Individual ticks may be removed by gentle traction, but it is important to take care and not separate the head from the body in doing so. The common insecticides mentioned in connection with lice are all effective against ticks, but are dependent on availability and subject to modern drug control regulations. At the time of going to press (1995) these regulations are subject to review.

Among those ectoparasites discussed in this chapter, fleas and lice are classified as *Insecta*, mites and ticks are *Arachnida*. The distinction between them is that insects have three body segments, three pairs of legs, wings and antennae; arachnids have two body segments, four pairs of legs in the adult and no wings or no antennae.

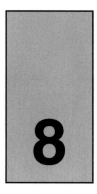

# 8 Bacterial and Fungal Diseases

The skin acts as an ideal medium for many bacterial organisms, as well as fungi and other parasites. By and large this does not lead to active infection, except perhaps where there is an underlying weakness that disturbs the balance between host and organism. Most bacteria on the skin live a commensal existence, meaning they cause no harm while deriving their existence from natural waste matter.

Bacterial infections may follow injection, abrasion, wounds, maceration (caused by prolonged wetting or topical skin treatment), harness sores, bites and foreign bodies.

## Rain Scald

Caused by *Dermatophilus congolensis*, rain scald is not uncommon in horses. Infection is dependent on the organism gaining access to broken skin, through which it invades. Spread may occur through the medium of insects, by direct contact between horses or through tack or common surfaces horses rub against. The infection may originate from carrier animals that harbour the organism without showing symptoms of the disease. *D. congolensis* is capable of forming spores which persist for long periods on the skin. Moisture is an essential part of the scenario as *D. congolensis* requires debilitated tissue as a medium on which to multiply. In other words, the health of the skin is weakened before clinical infection occurs.

### Clinical Signs

Matted areas of hair reveal small, circular, moist lesions when removed.

If these run together they may produce large denuded areas of skin. The exposed skin is inflamed, bearing a moist discharge and is raw-looking.

As the name rain scald implies, the areas of the horse affected are those that get wet when a horse is exposed to constant rain and lesions tend to follow the pattern of rain draining naturally from the horse's back. Other expressions of the disease may occur on isolated areas of the horse's anatomy that are permanently wet for one reason or another, such as the legs and face for example. Thus, they may occur on the legs of a horse standing permanently in wet conditions or on the face of a horse whose head is constantly over the door in the rain. Lesions occurring on white areas of skin may confuse the diagnosis with that of photosensitisation.

## Diagnosis

The appearance of rain scald is fairly typical and the organism can be isolated from samples taken from affected areas. It may also be cultured directly from skin lesions. Probably the most significant diagnostic factor is the pattern the gross lesions take which relates directly to the flow of water on the skin.

## Control and Treatment

It is essential that the animal be protected from the source of its problem, be that rain, and so on. Effective treatment involves removal of the scabs and use of mild disinfectants like dilute chlorhexidine to destroy the organism. In severe cases antibiotics may be needed by injection, the drug of choice being penicillin, either alone or in combination with streptomycin. These should be used for not less than five days.

# Greasy Heel or Mud Fever

As the name implies, greasy heel is a condition that occurs at the back of the lower limb. It is also caused by *Dermatophilus* organisms. It is particularly significant in non-pigmented areas, especially on horses kept in wet or unhygienic conditions. Secondary invasion of lesions with other bacteria is not uncommon.

## Clinical Signs

The predominant sign is weeping from the skin and as the condition

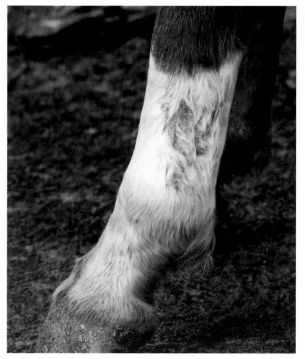

*Mud fever lesion on a horse's cannon*

develops there is fissure development, loss of hair, and extreme tenderness in the area. Secondary bacterial infection exacerbates the symptoms and the affected area may be raw and painful to the touch.

## Diagnosis

The condition is not difficult to diagnose if the typical signs are seen with a detectable association to wet underfoot conditions or unhygienic stables. It may be confused with other forms of dermatitis (for example, mange) and where the condition is unresponsive to treatment, scrapings may need to be taken for laboratory examination.

## Control and Treatment

The first requirement of treatment is to eliminate the underlying cause. Wet bedding must be removed and standards of management improved to ensure the animal is not standing in wet or dirty conditions. It may be necessary to clip the affected area and apply antiseptics or local antibiotic preparations to kill any secondary infection. It is important to remove scabs beneath which organisms can find protection. In obdurate cases with severe skin reaction and swelling of the limb, antibiotics may need to be given by parenteral injection. Local anti-inflammatory agents may also be of help in conjunction with antibiotics in some particularly aggravated situations.

Control of this condition means keeping animals out of wet or unhygienic standing conditions. After exercise, the horse's legs should be washed and dried thoroughly; wounds or abrasions should be treated with antiseptics and protected from possible infection with a suitable ointment.

Horses with mud fever should not be turned out in conditions which will only perpetuate symptoms.

# Folliculitis

This is the name given to infection of the hair follicles. It occurs when organisms gain access to the follicles, perhaps as a result of insect bites for example. It is recognised as pimples or pustules within the substance of the skin that can generally be picked up between the fingers and are usually painful when pinched.

Folliculitis may be caused by organisms like *Staphylococcus* and may advance to furunculosis (boils). *Streptococcus equi* and *Streptococcus zooepidemicus* can cause similar lesions.

## Clinical Signs

Lesions may occur where there is pressure from tack, and this may be associated with severe sweating. The critical factor is probably the effect of friction together with the elimination of air during the period of exercise-induced sweating leading to invasion of the follicles with bacteria.

A similar condition may occur on the back of the pastern and fetlock and is distinct from greasy heel.

Lesions may also appear on the tail as a consequence of rubbing, which, as we have already seen, results from a number of different causes, particularly sweet itch.

## Diagnosis

Infecting organisms may be isolated from lesions and cultured for identification and sensitivity purposes. This can be achieved by releasing the pus from an infected follicle by pricking it with a needle.

## Control and Treatment

Antibiotics may be needed for several days, depending on the organism and the response achieved. Selection of drug is best based on the result of a sensitivity test. Topical treatment with suitable dilute antiseptic or disinfectant solutions may help, as may surface treatment with selected antibiotic ointments.

# Abscess and Deeper Infection

Deeper infection of skin structures includes abscesses, fistulae, which generally indicate the presence of embedded foreign matter, and boils (furunculosis), which may rupture and release their contained pus to the exterior.

Abscesses are areas of pus accumulation due to infection with a variety of bacterial organisms (often mixed), and are marked by the development of a lining that contains the pus and restricts its release into neighbouring tissues. An abscess may form around a foreign body that gains access to a localised area, being generated by organisms that enter with it. Thus, abscesses may form around such objects as thorns, grit, or as a result of parasite larvae (although granulomas are more likely to develop here).

Treatment involves application of poultices to draw the abscess, or surgical drainage together with lavage of the abscess cavity with solutions such as hydrogen peroxide and other suitable antiseptics. Local treatment is always preferable where an abscess is close to the surface. The difficulty with parenteral antibiotic treatment is the nature of the abscess and the problem the drug has in coming into contact with the offending organism in these situations. Effectively, the pus protects the organism and creates the possibility of resistance.

In conditions like *Rhodococcus equi* infection of foals, abscesses tend to develop in areas, like the lungs and bowel, where they cannot easily be reached by surgical means. In these cases, antibiotics may be the only line of treatment available and the treatment period may extend for many weeks.

Abscess formation occurs as routine in strangles, a bacterial disease caused by *Streptococcus equi*. These abscesses form in the lymphatic glands at the lower side and back of the jaw and they normally burst and discharge outwardly, the discharged material being infectious on contact surfaces for as long as six weeks.

Treatment with antibiotics is inadvisable in most cases and recovery is usually complete after the glands have opened and drained fully.

# Cellulitis

A more serious occurrence is the development of cellulitis, where a bacterial infection spreads under the skin and follows the path of least resistance.

This type of eventuality can be very difficult to stop and is often precipitated by the subcutaneous injection of irritant drugs or as a result of the introduction of organisms in the course of routine injection. Such a possibility indicates the need for extreme care and accentuates the demand for skin sterility whenever and however an injection is given. A particular problem is that infections introduced in this way may contain a mixture of organisms. Treatment may therefore be difficult and it is not unknown for horses to die as a result of cellulitis.

Affected horses may have a raised temperature and be off food. However, the infection may spread at such a rate that there is little time for bacterial isolation; antibiotic treatment may need to be instituted empirically to begin with.

Results are often fruitless and there is nothing worse than helplessly watching an animal die from this type of infection.

# Ulcerative Lymphangitis

This condition is most common in the hind limb and is a bacterial infection caused by a variety of organisms, for example, *Corynebacterium pseudotuberculosis* or *Rhodococcus equi*. The infection gains access through cuts or abrasions on the lower limb and is most likely to occur where horses are kept in unhygienic conditions.

## Clinical Signs

The affected limb is swollen and painful to the touch. The horse is very likely to have a raised temperature. Nodules may be detected under the skin in the region of the fetlock and cannon. These nodules may enlarge and rupture to discharge green pus. The lymphatic vessels are involved and there is a tendency to weeping from the skin with abscess and ulcer formation along the course of these vessels.

The lower limb may remain permanently enlarged after the condition has been resolved.

## Diagnosis

A definite diagnosis will depend on the isolation of one of the organisms from sample material taken from the infected limb. The condition will have to be distinguished from other causes of leg filling which may be sterile in nature, for example, oedema.

## Control and Treatment

Ulcerative lymphangitis is not a very common condition today but, being caused by bacteria, it is treated preferably by antibiotics which are selected on the basis of sensitivity tests.

However, time may not allow for delay in instigating treatment but it should be remembered that *R. equi* in particular can be highly resistant and treatment can be needed for protracted periods. It is therefore essential to begin antibiotic treatment at the earliest possible stage where infection is detected and this must be done with broad-spectrum cover until tests can decide on a specific antibiotic if this fails.

It is vital to ensure stable hygiene and dietary factors as well as regular exercise are important in preventing relapses.

# Acne

Acne, or Canadian horsepox is a bacterial skin disease also caused by *Corynebacterium pseudotuberculosis* and is commonly seen in areas which come in contact with tack, like the saddle and girth. It is marked by small pustules and antibiotics may be required to ensure recovery.

# Bacterial Granuloma

A granuloma is a tumour-like mass of granulation tissue, varing in size from that of a pea upwards (like proud flesh in appearance). It is often provoked by the intrusion of a foreign body and marks the development of an infectious response to its presence. Treatment is difficult as antibiotics (because of the nature of the lesion) may have difficulty reaching the offending organism and resistance is the common result. Besides, if there is a foreign body present this will have to be removed. The essence of treatment in any such case is to surgically remove the offending tissue and to control infection with suitable antibiotics as the surrounding tissues repair.

Actinomycotic mycetoma is a similar type of lesion caused by the organisms *Nocardia* and *Actinomyces*.

## Skin Tuberculosis

Skin tuberculosis is a condition that is commonly seen in cattle. It can occur in horses. It is represented by small painful lumps on the abdomen and limbs, usually on the path of lymphatic vessels.

## Glanders

Glanders is an uncommon condition (last reported in 1928 in the UK) caused by *Actinobacillus mallei*. The condition is marked by respiratory nodule development and skin lesions (referred to as farcy) that discharge highly infectious pus.

Glanders is often fatal in horses, but has a particular importance because of being transmissible to humans. The mallein test is an intradermal test carried out for glanders.

## Ringworm

The most common fungal skin infection of horses is ringworm. It has a major significance in equine skin disease but is also important in being transmissible to humans who come in contact with some of the causal organisms. The fungus which is responsible for most equine ringworm is *Trichophyton equinum*. Other species of *Trichophyton* as well as species of *Microsporum* may also be implicated. A significant factor is that spores of these fungi can survive for months off a host, and that they are easily spread by direct contact, human transmission and by means of fomites (described as inanimate objects capable of carrying disease, examples of which are faeces, tack, implements, bedding). Species of

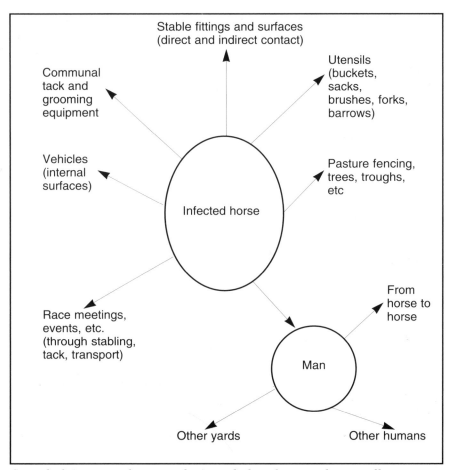

Stable fittings and surfaces
(direct and indirect contact)

Utensils
(buckets,
sacks,
brushes, forks,
barrows)

Communal
tack and
grooming
equipment

Vehicles
(internal
surfaces)

Pasture fencing,
trees, troughs,
etc

Infected horse

From
horse to
horse

Race meetings,
events, etc.
(through stabling,
tack, transport)

Man

Other yards

Other humans

*Spread of ringworm: how transfer is made from horse and eventually to man*

fungus which affect other animals are generally transmissible and horses may be infected from contact with cattle, sheep or goats, but rodents might also be implicated in some situations, as may dogs and cats.

Some species of fungus (for example, *Microsporum gypseum*), are normal soil inhabitants and may gain access to horses from this source. It may then spread from an individual infected animal.

Fungi that cause ringworm can only live on the surface of the skin and cannot penetrate through to living tissues or exist on open skin areas, like wounds or sores. The infection also only influences actively growing hair and this is why there is a tendency for the lesions to adopt the circular

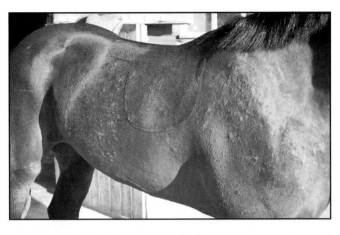

*Ringworm lesions caused by* Trichophyton equinum

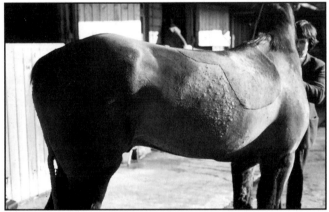

*The same horse from a different angle*

pattern they do, spreading outwardly from a central core; a detail that probably explains the origin of the name.

Infection is influenced by the health of the host animal but also by such factors as prevalent temperatures and the influence of tack, and sweating, on the microclimate of individual areas of skin. Infection often exposes an underlying weakness in the defensive mechanisms of the infected animal, which may occur for many reasons. Malnutrition is an obvious factor, as is age, because of the influence on immunity (immature in youth, declining in age). The level of exposure also counts as active infection on an animal tends to increase the disease risk for others and this leads to a probable increase in virulence of the infection.

## Clinical Signs

A practical reality in dealing with skin diseases is that lesions of different conditions may appear similar on gross examination and only the demon-stration of an organism or parasite might finally decide the diagnosis. However, having said that, the lesions in ringworm are very typical having a circular, radiant appearance and loss of hair with scaling of the skin. The condition is also highly infectious, spreading easily when ignored, mainly by means of human contact and through the medium of grooming equipment, tack, field posts, and so on. Horses do not tend to scratch at lesions, although they can be sensitive to the touch. However, it must be realised that these infections are readily transmitted to humans and people dealing with infected horses need to take care. Lesions that come in contact with tack (for example, the girth), can be very irritable and result in raw denuded areas that are extremely sensitive to touch.

Plucked hair over ringworm lesions leave grey glistening skin which scales over in one to two days.

*Microsporum* infections often occur after fly bites. Lesions are smaller than *Trichophyton* lesions, and the scabs less easy to remove.

Frequently ringworm occurs after the horse has travelled to shows, race meetings, competitions, and so on; lesions are seen in one to two weeks. Infection may be spread on the affected horse through grooming as well as being spread between horses from the same source where common tack or equipment are in use.

## Diagnosis

Ringworm lesions can occur on most parts of the body. They commonly appear on the face and neck, but where spread has occurred through grooming equipment they may appear on any part of the body, each between about 12 mm to 25 mm in diameter.

Other more chronic skin lesions may cause confusion in diagnosis (for example, sarcoids), but the rate of their appearance and the nature of spread will indicate the cause. For specific diagnosis, skin scrapings or biopsies are taken and these are examined in a suitably equipped labora-tory where the infecting fungus may be identified.

## Control and Treatment

As ringworm varies in its extent and clinical effect, treatment will depend on the degree of infection. Effectively, there are two approaches: local or oral treatment.

Local treatment consists of drugs applied as washes (which may be used over large areas) or those applied to individual lesions by means of sprays, paints or ointments. Oral treatment is with drugs such as griseofulvin.

Some mild infections may regress without treatment while others are very slow to respond.

There is a need to take immediate action to prevent further spread, to halt contamination of the local environment as well as any fomite that might extend the problem. This involves disinfection of stables as well as infected animals to reduce the possibility of future ringworm development. Suspect bedding should be burned, walls and other surfaces washed down with washing soda or household bleach (sodium hypochlorite). It is possible for horses to become re-infected with the disease within about eight weeks of clearing up an initial infection.

Drugs for local lesion treatment are numerous and include miconazole and trichlorophen (topical fungicide) which are both useful, often in spray form. Washes that include natamycin are very effective, but solutions containing chlorhexidine may prove helpful in early cases.

Orally, griseofulvin is the drug of choice, although the response may sometimes be slow and treatment required over an extended period of time (at least seven to ten days). It is also suggested that in-foal mares should not be treated with this drug because of the possibility of causing developmental problems in the foal.

## Other Fungal Infections

In addition to *Trichophyton* and *Microsporum, Candida albicans* is another fungal organism occasionally isolated from skin condtions in horses. It is a natural inhabitant of the digestive and reproductive tracts. It will usually only cause skin disease after skin has been weakened by constant wetting or where there is lowered resistance for other reasons. Treatment is usually effected by removing the underlying cause, but local or systemic treatment with drugs such as nystatin (locally or systemically), miconazole or clotrimazole (locally), or ketoconazole and amphotericin B (systemically) may be used.

*Aspergillus* species as well as many other species of fungus may be identified from skin lesions and treatment in each case will depend on identification of the organism and use of a drug to which it is sensitive. There is also a need to correct underlying resistance problems that allow normally harmless organisms to become associated with disease.

Fungi may develop in granulomas and abscess-type developments involving deeper skin structures. The basis for treatment is to flush or dissect the abscess and treat the organisms with suitable antifungals where this is possible.

It should be appreciated that aside from ringworm, these other fungal conditions are not common and usually seen only in isolated cases. Horses do not normally become infected on a herd basis, and there is little risk of transmission from one animal to another under normal circumstances.

A fungal infection that may be confused with lymphangitis, sporotrichosis may spread internally. Identification of this and most other fungi is a specialist function and best carried out by suitably equipped laboratories. The condition will respond to modern antifungal drugs when caught in its early stages. However, internal spread seriously influences the prognosis.

It is also possible that injured or debilitated tissues in any part of the body will become colonised by fungi, especially in the wake of antibiotic treatment where the underlying tissue is still unhealthy. This is quite common in areas like the respiratory and reproductive tracts.

Effective drugs for systemic use are ketoconazole and amphotericin B.

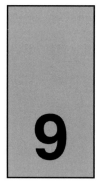

# 9 Allergies and Poisons

An allergy is a reaction that occurs as a result of meeting with an antigen (an antigen being any substance which is capable of inducing an immune response, causing the production of an antibody). It is generally a hypersensitivity to substances met within the environment. Antigens are composed of foreign proteins, like bacteria, parasites, fungi, viruses, and so on. However, this is an over-simplification as any of these organisms will have many constituent parts which are capable of being antigenic.

Allergic skin conditions may occur as a response to allergens inhaled (such as plant pollens, moulds, dust mites) and clinical symptoms will vary with availabilitiy of the allergen, be that seasonal or otherwise. There is skin irritation with multiple eruptions, hair loss and the pattern of the reaction will suggest that the condition is systemic rather than local.

## Management of Allergies

Localised allergies are epitomised by sweet itch, while there is some suggestion that exercise induced pulmonary haemorrhage (EIPH) is in some cases associated with allergic reactions of the respiratory system.

Systemic allergens, to be significant, must be light enough to be airborne and sufficiently small to gain access to the respiratory tract. This eliminates most flower pollens, although many allergenic pollens have not yet been identified. Birch, oak, elm, maple, ash, conifer, are all prospective sources of pollen which tends to appear at specific times of the year, and there are many others.

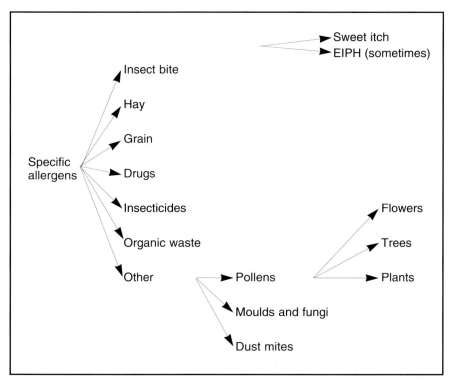

*Allergic conditions. Pollen counts are high on warm, dry days, and low on cold, wet days*

Plant pollens are released mainly during the morning and are influenced by weather conditions, being lowest on cold, wet days, highest on dry, warm days. They are inevitably at their most available during the months of plant growth and are released at some or all phases of the growing season depending on species.

Pollens from rape-seed have been reported to be a cause of allergenic respiratory disease in horses, although the case has yet to be satisfactorily proven. The idea that whole yards of horses can be affected at the same time is unlikely and the more probable reality is that intercurrent infection is also present.

Moulds and fungi are available at all times of the year and their spores are sufficiently small for them to be carried in large numbers in the air and to be able to gain access to tissues where they can cause allergies. These organisms can grow on many types of medium, including soil, inside stables, on hay or straw, on cereals, grasses, rotten materials, organic waste, and are often dense in inhaled air. Some tolerate high temperatures. Examples we encounter in our daily lives are organisms growing on waste food, within refrigerators, on damp surfaces and so on.

The allergenic propensities of dust are usually dependent on the presence within it of mites, similar to the situation with human house mite allergy. However, *Dermatophagoides*, the most common mite associated with equine dust allergies is unable to survive on disinfected surfaces or in areas of high humidity.

## Clinical Signs

The first sign of allergy is due to the cellular reaction within the respiratory system resulting from contact with an allergen. There is serum effusion and localised inflammation resulting in closure of small bronchioles. This results in reduced oxygen uptake from the lungs and causes an immediate increase in respiratory rate and effort.

Local allergic reactions will be similar to those experienced in connection with insect bites, and responses to the saliva and faeces of mange mites. The intense irritation in sweet itch is frequently a result of allergy developed against the bite of *Culicoides* species.

Marked eyelid oedema occurs and is sometimes seen after the introduction of new hay. Skin wheals may appear when new grain is introduced to the diet. Other similar reactions may ensue with allergies to drugs like penicillin, or to insecticides, or chemicals and so on.

## Diagnosis

Diagnosis is not always simple and depends on identification of the causative allergen.

The only specific way of determining this is through intradermal skin tests, and it is vital that animals being tested are not under the influence of any drug which might affect the test (for example, cortisone). The allergens suspected of causing the disease are injected into the skin in tiny amounts. The response to their presence is evaluated after some 15 to 30 minutes, by measuring the skin reaction and comparing it with the reaction of a control substance (for example, saline), which will produce no reaction.

It has to be appreciated that positive reactions only indicate the animal is sensitive to the substance causing it; there are false positive and false negatives and a great deal of objective thought has to be put into the interpretation of results. Pitfalls can arise through failures in technique and through faults in the test materials or through their contamination with any kind of irritant substance.

## Control

While a certain degree of success is achieved by controlling the environment of stabled horses to limit respiratory allergens, success is decided by the type of allergen and how it might gain access to the afflicted horse. Pollen allergens travel on the wind and thus gain access to air even in enclosed areas; however, keeping affected horses indoors may reduce exposure. Weather conditions are an important element in this disease; warm air and sunshine are factors adversely affecting sufferers, although spores from moulds and their like may be more common at night.

Bedding and hay are common sources of moulds and it is possible that particular types of buildings may bear high spore counts, though this might well be reduced with effective cleaning and hygiene. Prevention of moisture and humidity build-up is therefore important and ventilation may be a key factor in reducing the proliferation of moulds and fungi.

The control of dust within stabling requires thought and attention to detail. Regular cleaning is important as well as strict quality control of hay and straw. It is also important to stir up as little dust as possible while horses are stabled and to keep walls and ceilings free of dust and cobwebs. These may harbour allergens that become agitated into the air when exposed to airflows, or even the effect of a horse clearing its nose or coughing.

## Treatment

Treatment is not a simple matter, especially as the condition is life-lasting and the most successful prevention is in keeping the animal free of the allergen. Difficult as this may seem, there is no doubt that efforts to clean up stable environment and eliminate evident sources (like dusty hay and straw) are often very beneficial.

Corticosteroids are sometimes used when symptoms are severe, but there are undesireable side-effects, as already stated. Resistance to infection is lowered; laminitis is also a possible side result. However, the principle consequence of long-term use is atrophy of the adrenal glands which can effect production of hydrocortisone, an important hormone involved in normal anti-inflammatory processes within the body.

The prime consideration in corticosteroid use is to keep treatment to a minimum and to withdraw use at the earliest possible time relative to symptoms. As a rule, however, these drugs should be a last choice and other drugs used wherever possible as an alternative.

Histamine is a byproduct of the allergic reaction which causes inflammation and is countered with varying degrees of success by the use of antihistamines. High dosage rates and expense are factors in using these drugs which may be needed for lengthy periods of time.

Clenbuterol is used with some success in respiratory allergies as it promotes bronchiole dilatation and aids the clearance of mucus from the lungs. The drug may disappoint in advanced cases.

Sodium cromoglycate is used by inhalation through a nebuliser for four consecutive days and though it is primarily recommended as a preventive it frequently provides relief for horses with chronic obstructive pulmonary disease (COPD).

Immunotherapy is a form of treatment whereby the animal is injected against an identified allergen in gradually increasing doses. The disadvantage is that a successful response is slow to develop, perhaps up to a year, and results can be disappointing. Other treatment may be necessary during the time injections are given in order to relieve the symptoms. Allergen extracts are given by subcutaneous injection and the increasing dose regime is designed to prevent any anaphylactic reaction. Animals under treatment are monitored after injection and any adverse response is treated on an emergency basis, though treatment will be continued as a rule. In mild cases, antihistamine therapy may be adequate, but treatment for shock may be necesary where the reaction is acute.

Failure of this kind of therapy arises when an animal is sensitive to a range of allergens, or where an animal has become sensitive to new allergens.

## Urticaria/Angioedema

Urticaria is a condition of the skin marked by the appearance of raised wheals which are frequently intensely itchy. They are caused by either an immune reaction or by direct contact with some chemicals. The condition is also sometimes known as nettle rash. The wheals may vary in size from 1–5 cm in diameter and the skin is not usually broken except by scratching. The reaction occurs following damage to the blood vessels of the skin.

Angioedema is a similar type reaction occurring in the tissues beneath the skin or mucous membranes. While there may or may not be itchiness, the lesions usually cover large areas and are generally painless.

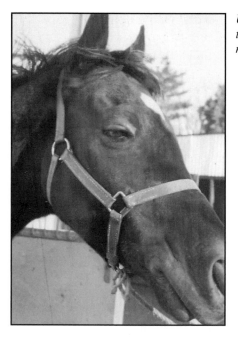

*Urticarial lesions on the head. Note the swollen eyelid, lips and nostril*

The causes are similar and may represent a reaction to parasites such as *Culicoides* or *Onchocerca* also to particular bacteria, drugs or food; or the condition might occur as a reaction to more than one of these substances at a time. Inhaled allergens may also play a part.

## Clinical Signs

There is reddening and development of oedema (fluid) beneath the skin. Depending on the severity of the reaction there may be a rise in body

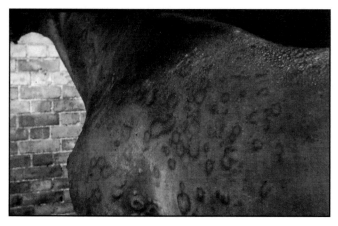

*Urticarial lesions on the body are raised and often intensely itchy*

temperature and lesions may be confined to areas like the face and abdomen or be more generalised. Oedema of the larynx may occur and this, inasmuch as it could compromise air intake, might prove very dangerous.

## Diagnosis

The nature of the reaction will suggest a diagnosis of urticaria/angiodedema, but detecting the precise cause may be difficult.

## Treatment

It will be necessary to treat the symptoms and alleviate tissue reactions in acute cases. It is vital, where possible, to detect and remove the causative factor as well, but drugs like antihistamines may have a useful part to play in immediate therapy as well as anti-inflammatory drugs which may be essential depending on the extent of the tissue reactions.

# Food Allergies

Food allergies are not that common in horses but where they do occur they are considered to be protein related. They may be caused by particular types of grass (for example, some clovers), also weeds like St. John's wort.

## Clinical Signs

The most common sign is of skin irritation though changes in the tissues of the digestive tract may cause diarrhoea, increased gas production and tail-scratching. Asthmatic-type changes in the respiratory system may also be seen.

## Diagnosis

Specific diagnosis can be very difficult. It may even be necessary to devise a diet free of all those substances which a horse has previously eaten in order to detect the offending substance. Each item may then be reintroduced to the diet individually until symptoms recur. The search

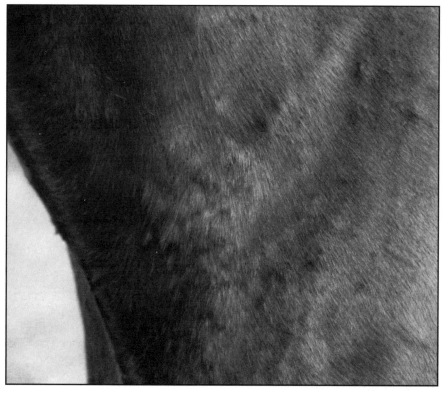

*Typical reaction on the horse's neck seen in food allergy*

will have to be painstaking and the ultimate answer is to keep the animal away from the material to which it is allergic.

Treatment will be on the same basis as for any other allergy.

## Contact Dermatitis

Allergic contact dermatitis results from substances which might come into contact with a horse's skin, like leather, plastic, fibre, various drugs and medications, parasiticides, insect repellants, and even types of bedding.

This condition has to be distinguished from non-allergic contact dermatitis. The latter is a result of substances like some anti-fungals or disinfectants used locally, or chemicals with which an animal may have come in contact over a period of time and which cause similar lesions.

## Clinical Signs

A critical factor is that the skin reaction seen is confined to the area that comes in contact with the allergen. Thus, lesions may be seen over an area treated with a substance, for example, beneath the saddle, girth or other tack, or over a whole area covered by a rug or blanket.

Lesions consist of small skin eruptions and it should be realised that broken areas of skin may in some of these cases become infected with bacteria, fungi and their like to further exacerbate the clinical situation.

## Diagnosis

Specific diagnosis is not easily achieved except by detecting the cause through direct observation and by response to its removal. Patch tests may be a practical prospect in the future, but are not yet adequately developed for use in the horse. These tests involve the use of test substances which are applied to the shaved skin using retaining patches. The reaction is gauged at 24-hour intervals for a period of three days.

## Treatment

The most effective therapy is to avoid the allergen.

Local anti-inflammatory drugs may be required to settle the horse's skin reaction, though their effect is purely palliative and can have no long-term benefit if the cause persists.

The same applies to any form of contact dermatitis: remove the cause and treat the lesions where this is necessary.

# Other Causes

Contact dermatitis may also arise from substances such as mustard blisters which cause swelling and scale formation; mercurial blisters also cause severe dermatitis. Severe blisters can cause alopecia, hypopigmentation and scar formation. They can also cause damage to the mouth and ulcers of the tongue (when licked).

Over-strength insecticides cause pruritis, dermatitis, alopecia, scarring and excoriation.

Scalding might occur on the navel from using iodine that was too strong; also from body excreta or discharges (for example, faecal, urinary, uterine or chronic wound discharges).

# Poisons

While most external poisons enter the body through the digestive tract and exert their influence on tissues they encounter either within that tract or by absorption into the systemic circulation, skin conditions are an essential diagnostic element of some. Inevitably this means a more chronic development of symptoms than would happen in acute poisoning where tissue destruction is likely to lead to early death.

Some poisons as sources of skin disease are discussed below.

## Aflatoxin

Aflatoxin is produced by the fungal organism, *Aspergillus flavus*, and is most commonly traced to contaminated grain or groundnut. The toxin is harmful to liver cells and also has an adverse effect on the immune system. Acute cases are marked by the appearance of blood at the nostrils and rectum, followed by convulsions and, very often, death. More chronic cases display anorexia, anaemia, jaundice, nervous signs, and roughness of the coat.

Diagnosis is based on symptoms as well as isolation of the toxin from contaminated feed. Treatment is symptomatic, using activated charcoal to protect the bowel and parenteral feeding combined with drugs to foster the repair of damaged liver tissue.

## Arsenic

Arsenic was commonly used as a stimulant for horses in the past. It may still appear as a constituent of weedkillers or fruit-tree sprays and is found in industrial waste.

Thickening of the skin may occur with hair loss (especially mane and tail) and broken skin is open to secondary infection. These are symptoms of chronic, low-grade poisoning. The more acute symptoms of high-level intake are mainly systemic and vary from abdominal pain to paralysis and blindness.

Arsenical poisoning is diagnosed on the basis of symptoms, history (confirming access to arsenical products) and can be confirmed on examination of kidney or liver sections. Sodium thiosulphate is used in treatment but success will depend on degree of intake and the damage done to vital organs.

## Ergot

Ergot is a product of the fungus, *Claviceps purpurea*, which may develop in the seed heads of grasses like rye grass, usually in the warmer months of the year.

Toxins produced cause constriction of blood vessels which may lead to tissue necrosis and gangrene. Areas affected are the extremities, ears, feet and tail. These may become cold and sections may slough off. Similar lesions may occur in some acute bacterial infections and in frostbite.

Diagnosis depends on symptoms and identification of the causative agent.

Treatment involves local treatment of affected parts, the use of drugs to promote circulation as well as removal of affected animals from crops contaminated by the fungus.

A further preventive measure is to top pastures at a stage before the seed heads develop.

## St John's wort

*Hypericum perfoliatum*, or as it is more usually known as, St John's wort, is a plant that occurs commonly in hedgerows and rough grazing.

Photosensitisation occurs in *Hypericum* poisoning and there is inflammation and necrosis of skin in white areas, which slough off. This process essentially involves the presence of a photodynamic agent (normally a breakdown product of chlorophyll) which accumulates under the skin and reacts to sunlight to bring about the disease process seen. Non-pigmented areas of skin are most susceptible and it is not uncommon for lesions to be confined to white areas only.

There is no specific treatment for this condition except to protect affected animals from direct sunlight, treat affected areas as for any similar type wound, encouraging skin regrowth and protecting exposed areas from infection and fly infestation. The outcome will be decided by the degree of the reaction and the extent of the white area affected. It is also essential to remove animals from the source of the photodynamic agent, if this can be identified.

Photosensitisation may also appear as a feature of ragwort (*Senecio jacoboea*) poisoning, a condition which is usually fatal. Numerous other plants and substances such as phenothiazine and sulfonamides may act as precipitating agents. It can also occur as a sequel to liver damage, in which case the primary cause of this damage needs to be addressed.

## Iodine Poisoning

Iodine poisoning is most commonly a result of prolonged oral treatment of animals for conditions such as ringworm with iodine containing drugs. Symptoms include skin scaling and hair loss; there may also be discharges from nose and eye. The diagnosis will be suggested by the history of iodine administration coupled with the symptoms. The first line of treatment is to remove the offending substance from the animal's intake.

## Mercury Poisoning

Mercury poisoning may occur as a result of absorption from the skin during blistering of horses with mercury containing compounds, or through ingestion of grain treated with mercurial insecticides. Symptoms include loss of hair in mane and tail, followed by a general loss of body hair. There is also gastroenteritis and emaciation. The local effect of mercury as a blister causes oedema, fissuring of the skin and painful local reaction. In case of poisoning, local affected areas should be cleaned off and an emollient ointment applied to the part. Any other source of mercury must be detected and removed.

## Pentachlorophenol

Pentachlorophenol is a wood preservative which sometimes gains access to shavings, sawdust or surfaces with which horses come into contact. It is also a constituent of waste oil.

There are early signs of contact dermatitis when the chemical comes in contact with the skin, but affected animals may also show systemic signs, including incoordination, loss of appetite and ultimate weight loss.

Removal of the offending material from the environment may require drastic measures if contact surfaces are heavily contaminated.

## Motor Oil

Motor oil can cause chronic inflammation of skin when used in conditions like sweet itch.

## Selenium Toxicity

Selenium toxicity occurs most commonly as a result of feeding excessive selenium supplements, although it can also occur as a consequence of eating food sources carrying high levels of the same substance. Some plants concentrate selenium and are therefore likely to lead to toxicity, other cases arise because of high soil levels.

Deficiencies arise in soils where selenium is found and thus not available to grazing animals.

Skin lesions only appear in cases of chronic poisoning as high intakes are responsible for acute fatalities. Aside from hair loss (mainly long hair of mane, tail and legs), a prominent sign of the condition is the development of hoof defects with cracking of horn and lameness. Affected animals lose condition, are lethargic and unable to perform to potential.

Diagnosis depends on the signs coupled with dietary evaluation and possibly blood tests and hair analysis.

Treatment involves removal of the source, although absorption can be reduced through dietary supplementation with copper. The correct dietary level of selenium is not less than 5ppm of dry matter. Levels in excess of 20ppm are associated with toxicity.

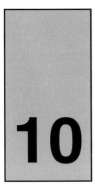

# 10 Tumours and Other Conditions

This chapter includes many conditions which, for one reason or another, are likely to be less well known to the average reader. It also includes conditions like warts, sarcoids and melanomas, all classified as tumours, which are among the most important skin conditions seen in horses.

We start with the tumours of skin and then look at the other conditions, which are arranged in alphabetical order to improve ease of access.

## Tumours of Skin

The main consideration with any form of skin tumour is its capacity to spread externally and through malignancy to ultimately attack internal organs (metastasize), with all the significance that has.

Tumours are thus either malignant or benign; however, benign tumours of the skin may pose problems for their owners because of their situation and nature, and this factor may ultimately be vital in deciding the soundness or otherwise of the horse. Sarcoids, for example, a form of skin tumour, may occur in areas where they will be interfered with by tack in ridden horses or appear on the mammary glands of mares where they pose particular problems when suckling a foal.

Basal cell tumours are benign growths that usually appear as solitary lumps in the neck and trunk region. They move freely under the skin and are not very common.

Fibromas are a similar type of benign growth that may be firm or soft in nature, the distinction only being made on microscopic examination of tissues from the lesion. Where necessary, they can be removed by surgery or by cryosurgery.

Fibromatosis is the condition where there are multiple fibromas. It also describes a more invasive form of skin tumour, which does not metastasize but is inclined to recur when removed.

Fibrosarcoma is a malignant form of fibroma. It develops as irregular skin lumps which are locally invasive, may ulcerate superficially, and are unlikely to metastasize. The only treatment is complete surgical excision.

Haemangioma is a benign tumour of blood vessels. It is well defined and coloured and occurs most commonly on the limbs. Haemangiosarcoma is the malignant form of the same condition and is highly invasive.

Haemangioendothelioma is an uncommon tumour found in the newborn. Lesions, located usually on the extremities, are poorly defined birthmarks which may ulcerate and become oedematous.

A keratoma is a benign tumour of the horn layer of the hoof. It is thought to occur as a consequence of irritation from the coronary band or sensitive laminae. The tumour creates a visible distortion of the hoof wall which may be associated with cracks and other growth defects. Intermittent lameness and periodic discharging fistulas are also a feature of the condition. Surgical removal is sometimes undertaken; however, complete regrowth of the excised hoof is slow and the condition is inclined to recur.

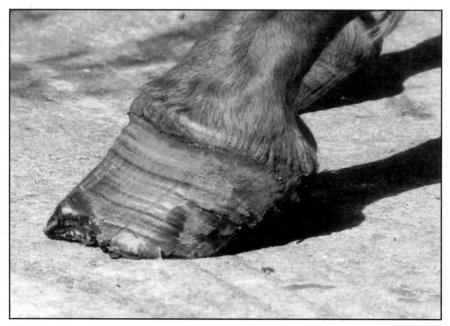

*The distortion on this foot was caused by a keratoma*

A lipoma is a benign tumour of the subcutaneous fat. It is circumscribed, soft to touch and may be seen on the neck and trunk. Diagnosis is confirmed on microscopic examination of tissue samples from the growth. These growths are not removed unless causing a problem.

Liposarcomas are the malignant form of the same growth but are rare in the horse.

Lymphosarcoma is a malignant tumour involving lymphocyte cells seen most commonly in middle-aged male horses. Growths may appear as hard skin nodules with associated hair loss and are capable of ulcerating. Local lymph nodes may enlarge and blood samples may show indications of leukaemia. The condition, being malignant, may spread to

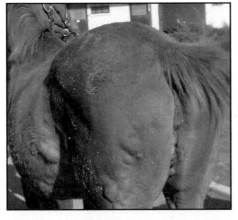

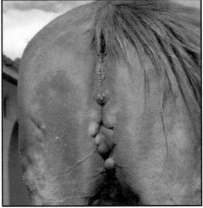

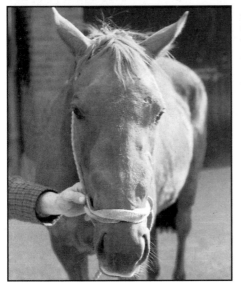

*Lymphosarcoma subcutis in a mare* (reading anticlockwise, from top right): *the clinical reaction in the perineal region; hind view, note the reactions under the skin; front view of mare*

other internal organs. Diagnosis is based on blood and local lesion analysis. The condition carries a poor prognosis and current treatment regimens in other species of animal are not usually considered practicable for horses.

Mast-cell tumours are small nodular masses which are generally benign (but potentially malignant) and are removed surgically where necessary; some regress spontaneously. They are seen about the eye, head and neck. Myxoma and myxosarcoma are other types of nodular tumour that occur only rarely in horses and which will only be diagnosed on the basis of microscopic examination.

Most of these tumours are removed surgically where this is thought necessary. However, where small growths are not interfering with the use of an animal it is often best to be conservative and not interfere unless there is a specific indication for doing so.

## Melanoma

Melanomas are tumours of the melanin-producing cells of the skin. They are relatively common in grey horses and can be benign or malignant. The incidence in greys increases with age. The most common sites are the perinaeum and sheath but tumours also appear around the eyelids (may occur on the third eyelid) and ears and sometimes in the upper jugular area of the neck.

*Melanomas on the perinaeum of a grey mare*

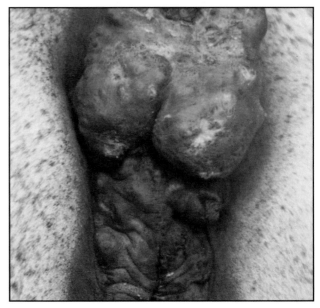

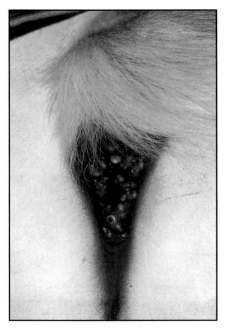

*Melanoma formation on the perinaeum of a gelding*

Most melanonas are small, well circumscribed nodules, likely to appear in clusters around the vulva and anus. They become increasingly common as grey horses age, but are seldom malignant or life-threatening, although the risk always exists. Tumours in the region of the vulva may complicate fertility by interfering with the vulvar seal and are a variable problem when mares are being covered and foaling.

Malignant melanomas are more likely to arise from mucous membrane rather than skin and are also likely to be ulcerated. The condition is usually progressive from the first appearance but this progress is generally slow.

Diagnosis is based on appearance combined with microscopic examination of tumour tissue when this becomes necessary on account of spread.

Treatment is surgical, either by direct excision or through the use of cryosurgery. Where metastasis has occurred, the prognosis for this condition is not good.

## Papillomas

A papilloma is a wart and papillomatosis is the name given to the disease state where there are a number of warts.

Warts are caused by viruses which are species specific and are the most common form of tumour seen in horses. They are usually multiple, more common in young animals and appear on the face, ears, genitalia and

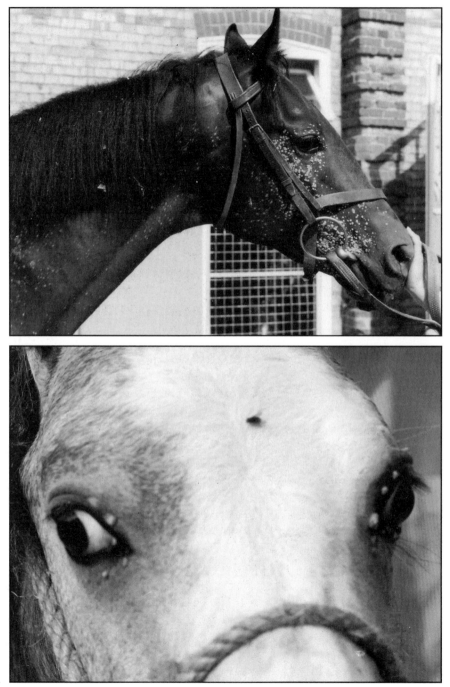

*Warts on a two-year-old horse* (top)*; they disappeared by the time the horse was three years old. Warts on the face* (above) *of a yearling colt*

under side of the body. They are often profuse about the mouth and muzzle. The virus is mainly transmitted by direct contact through tack, grooming equipment and by the medium of posts, fencing and stable surfaces. Foals may be infected when suckling their dams. The incubation period is believed to be in the region of two to three months. Papillomas can occur as a congenital disease in foals.

Aural plaques are a form of papillomatosis in the ear; they start as small papules that enlarge into hyperkeratotic plaques.

Diagnosis of warts is based on gross appearances as well as microscopic examination of affected tissue where this is felt necessary. Warts in older horses may be confused with similar looking types of sarcoid.

Most warts regress spontaneously, although the development of self-cure may take a prolonged time to occur. Sometimes autogenous vaccines are prepared from wart tissue in persistent cases but results are variable and commonly disappointing. The prepared vaccine is injected in 2ml doses at two-weekly intervals for three or four times.

Warts may be removed by cryosurgery or by treatment with caustic chemicals but these are potentially dangerous substances and must be used in skilled hands.

Where there are persistent problems with warts on a farm, disinfection of likely contact sources is a vital part of prevention.

## Sarcoid

Sarcoids are a very common, locally aggressive type of tumour in adult horses, thought to be viral in origin and appearing as single growths or multiple clusters, capable of growing to several centimetres in diameter and having several types in appearance. They occur on the head, neck, trunk, in the inguinal region and medial side of the upper hind limb most commonly. There are four described types:

1. Verrucous sarcoids are like warts, small and similar shaped, though they may be raw and bleeding or dry and scaly and generally free of hair.
2. Fibroblastic sarcoids are large and firm and may be dry and covered or ulcerated. These may on occasion be confused with granulation tissue, some types of infection or fibroma development and diagnosis will only be confirmed in these cases on microscopic examination of sarcoid tissue.
3. Mixed sarcoids are a combination of the first two types
4. Occult sarcoids are flat, slow-growing, scaly lesions that often appear on the face, ears and eyelids and which may later develop into the other types. They are also common about the scrotum, prepuce and udder.

*A fibroblastic sarcoid in the inguinal region*

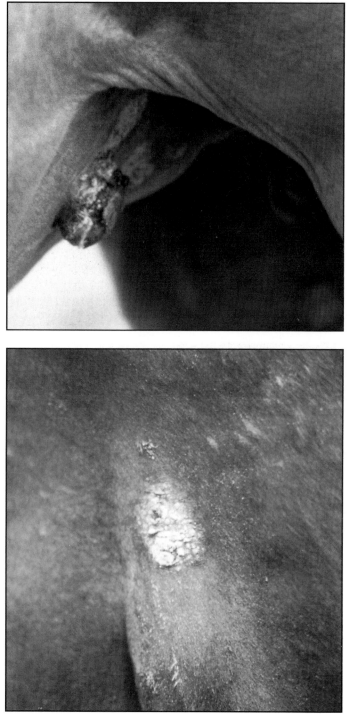

*A mixed sarcoid on the chest*

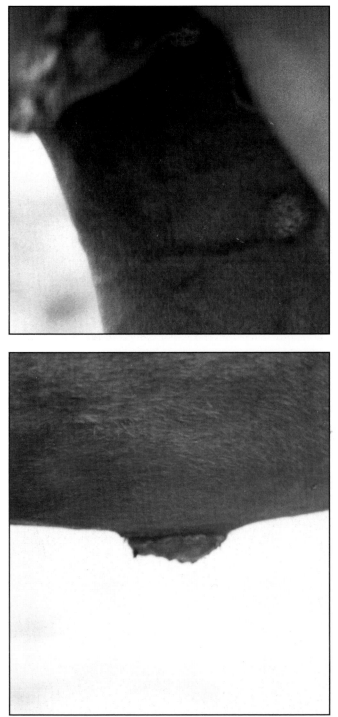

*An occult
sarcoid high on
the inner leg*

*Verrucous sarcoid
on the underside
of the belly*

Occasionally sarcoids will disappear spontaneously, but this is rare and most sarcoids are treated surgically, either by direct excision, or more commonly today with the use of cryosurgery (after which there may be scars and leukotrichia). Direct surgical interference sometimes leads to disappointment because of further growth of incompletely removed tumour tissue, whereas results using cryosurgery are considerably more satisfactory.

Various forms of immunotherapy have been tried with differing degrees of success. Reactions to the vaccines produced are sometimes severe and anaphylactic deaths have been reported in rare cases.

## Squamous Cell Carcinomas

An increasingly common form of skin tumour, squamous cell carcinomas (SCC) appear on the head, in the region of the eye and its close tissues, at junctions of mucous membrane and skin, on the penis and related organs of males and on the perinaeum of mares. These growths are locally invasive but may metastasize to other organs, like local lymph nodes and lungs. They appear as cauliflower-style growths or as active, ulcerative lesions that are covered with dried crusts. They frequently smell.

*Congenital skin tumour on a foal's head*

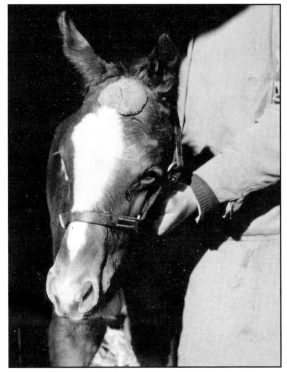

Diagnosis is confirmed by microscopic examination.

Treatment is surgical in early cases but the risk of internal spread in active, established lesions has to be considered, in which case the prognosis is poor. However, this does not mean that all horses with SCCs have to be viewed with such pessimism.

## Schwannomas

Schwannomas are benign tumours of young animals, originating in nervous tissue, and occurring mainly on the face and eyelids. They are surgically removed.

## Sebaceous Gland Tumours

Sebaceous gland tumours are not common and are often diagnosed as warts when they do occur. They are small nodules that are not connected to underlying tissues. Malignant forms are known to metastasize and tumours that are incompletely removed tend to regrow.

Seborrhoea means discharge of sebum and is not a common feature of equine skin conditions.

## Generalised Steatitis

Generalised steatitis is marked by ill-defined subcutaneous plaques, and has been associated with selenium deficiency.

## Sweat Gland Tumours

Sweat gland tumours are also uncommon but are sometimes seen on the ears and perinaeum. Malignant forms are known in other animals and surgical removal is advised when diagnosed on microscopic examination.

# Amyloidosis

Amyloidosis occurs as a primary or secondary condition, usually manifested by upper respiratory and/or skin disorder characterised by a prolonged, progressive course.

Skin lesions include wheals and nodules, seen in the head, neck and pectoral regions. Internal lesions occur secondary to chronic inflammation or vaccination.

The diagnosis of this condition is based on the animal's history, signs and biopsy.

## Anhidrosis

Anhidrosis is an inability to sweat. Sweating is the process which regulates body temperature and is responsible for 75 per cent of lost body heat. Anhidrosis is not affected by diet or electrolyte intake and is usually caused by a change from temperate to hot humid climates.

Symptoms are caused by failure of sweat production and include increased heart rate, dry skin, hair loss, inappetance, inability to perform athletically, and sometimes fever.

Diagnosis is based on the history and signs and is assisted by intradermal injections of adrenalin which provokes sweating in healthy animals.

The only form of reliable treatment is to provide a cooler and less humid environment, to wet the animal with water periodically, to exercise it during the cooler hours and acclimatise it gradually to warmer climatic conditions. Some animals may eventually have to be returned to their original conditions before normality is restored.

## Collagenolytic Granuloma

Collagenolytic granuloma (equine eosinophilic granuloma or EEG) is a common lesion in horses, seen more often in ponies, riding horses and eventers than Thoroughbreds or heavy horses.

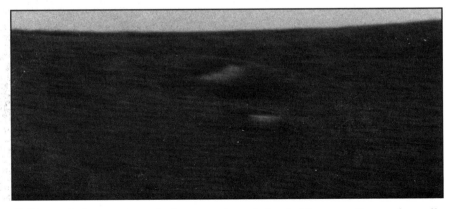

*Collagenolytic granuloma lesions on a horse's back. These are firm and usually painless to touch*

It is a non-pruritic, nodular skin condition of uncertain aetiology. It could be caused by hypersensitivity to insect bites. Lesions may be single or multiple and vary in size from 1 cm to 10cm; they are firm, well demarcated, and not painful. They are most common in the saddle area, neck, trunk and quarters and may become calcified in time.

Corticosteroid therapy has been used in some cases, either locally or systemically, but with only moderate success. Particular lesions can be removed surgically when required, especially if calcified and causing problems with tack.

## Ear Diseases

Diseases of the external ear (otitis externa) are common in horses and include bacterial, fungal and parasitic causes, allergy, pigment disorders, cancers and similar conditions.

The ear may also be involved in toxic conditions like ergot poisoning, also with pemphigus, lupus erythematosus and warts.

Aural plaques are non-irritant and occur on the inner surface of the ear, possibly due to a chronic reaction to blackfly bites; it is also suggested that they may be a form of wart.

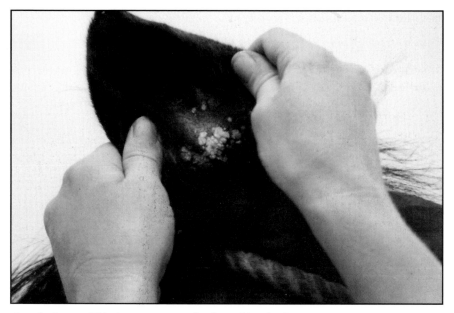

*Aural plaque. This horse was not bothered by the lesions on its ear*

Ear problems are usually associated with head shaking and affected horses resent their ears being touched. Diagnosis requires careful examination together with swabs for infectious causes or for the detection of mites.

(Cytology is the direct examination of prepared smears for cells and organisms and is a useful aid to diagnosis.)

Treatment requires the cleaning away of any offending material, like discharges, and care must be taken not to impact debris into the ear canal with the use of swabs. This can be achieved by flushing the external ear out with antiseptics or wax-removing substances like propylene glycol.

Specific drug use will depend on the cause, but corticosteroid containing drugs may be of use where there is acute tissue irritation. Solutions of vinegar in water are helpful in bacterial and fungal infections. Antibiotics may also be used systemically in some ear infections and are an advantage where pain limits local interference.

It must be appreciated that there is a risk in *any* interference involving the ear. No treatment should be undertaken except under veterinary advice.

## Fistulous Withers

Fistulous withers involves infection of the supraspinous bursa, the infection usually reaching the site from the general system, and is frequently considered to be associated with *Brucella abortus* organisms. The initial swelling can be extremely painful and lead to discharging tracts and fistulae which are difficult to clear up. Affected horses should have serum tests for *Brucella* organisms carried out because of the public health aspects of this infection. Affected horses respond better to *Brucella* vaccination than to any other form of therapy, although vaccinal reactions are known and there is always the possibility that other organisms are involved. However, there has been a significant drop in cases since bovine brucellosis has become controlled.

## Filling in the Legs

Filling in the legs is a term used to describe passive filling in stabled horses experiencing varying degrees of uniform oedema with obliteration of the normal anatomical outlines.

While the legs of horses confined to their boxes are likely to fill through lack of exercise, the condition is more commonly related to mild

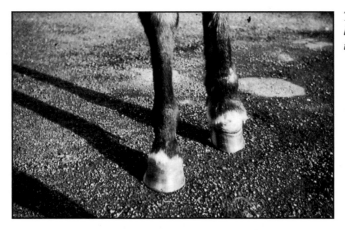

*The filling in this leg was caused by infection*

toxic conditions stemming from the bowel or similarly mild digestive upsets.

On a more serious note, circulatory problems may be the cause. It can also occur as a consequence of feed change or as a result of over-feeding. Filling is generally noted in the morning and may disappear with exercise. A single occurrence might not be of note but in competing animals may be accompanied by a reduction in the level of performance.

A critical factor is that filling is noted in more than one limb, very often all four. When only one limb is filled it is wise to consider an alternative cause (for example, infection). Laxatives or purgatives may be necessary to relieve the symptoms and there is little need to be excessive in this. The horse is then returned to a simple diet of hay and small quantities of oats.

Horses whose legs fill when fed on heavy concentrate diets should have the quantity reduced or the feed changed. Most legs fill after injuries and this distinct type of filling is associated with wounds and grazes. The cause is interference with normal limb circulation and takes longer to disappear, but need not always keep an animal out of work.

Where circulation is a cause, the situation is more serious and professional advice is needed to determine the soundness of the heart and other organs.

## Haematomas

Haematomas arise as collections of blood (usually clotted) beneath the skin. They result from local haemorrhage that might follow a kick or contusion of any kind. The tendency is for the blood to form a local swelling which may be as large as a football, depending on the amount of blood collected. Many of these swellings, especially in the front of the sternum, can be very large and take many weeks to disappear.

Treatment is usually inadvisable, although it may be necessary to distinguish between a haematoma and an abscess. However, the blood can act as an ideal medium for bacterial growth and care must be taken not to introduce infection by unwarranted intrusions into the area. Sternal haematomas tend to appear more commonly in backward yearlings, but the prognosis is good given patience and time for regression.

Once the haematoma has settled and the source of the bleeding has had time to heal, ultrasound may prove very effective in reducing the swelling. However, it must be appreciated that too early use of this equipment can cause resorption of a clot and provoke fresh bleeding.

Surgical drainage after clotting has occurred may speed resolution but the risk of infection favours a more conservative approach.

## Helminth Diseases

Skin diseases related to helminth parasites include cutaneous habronemiasis, also the irritation caused by *Onchocerca* and *Oxyuris*.

## Hereditary Diseases and Pigment Disorders

If present at birth, any hereditary disease condition is termed congenital; if appearing later it is said to be tardive.

Albinism is rare; horses have white skin and hair and lack pigment in the iris. Black hair follicular dysplasia occurs in Appaloosas, losing black hair in certain areas. The condition is considered, but is not proven to be, hereditary. Curly coat is a hereditary condition in Percherons.

Cutaneous asthenia is a condition in which there is skin fragility. It occurs as a hereditary condition in the Quarter Horse, in which affected skin may easily tear. It is due to a defect in collagen formation, or to its excessive degradation.

Dentigerous cysts appear at the base of the ear and contain embryonic teeth.

Epitheliogenesis imperfecta (or aplasia cutis) is a fatal hereditary condition in which there is absence of areas of skin.

Leukoderma is depigmentation after injury, perhaps a severe blister, with associated scarring. It occurs as depigmented areas of skin around the mouth and eyes, seen most commonly in Arab horses, and these lesions may be reversible.

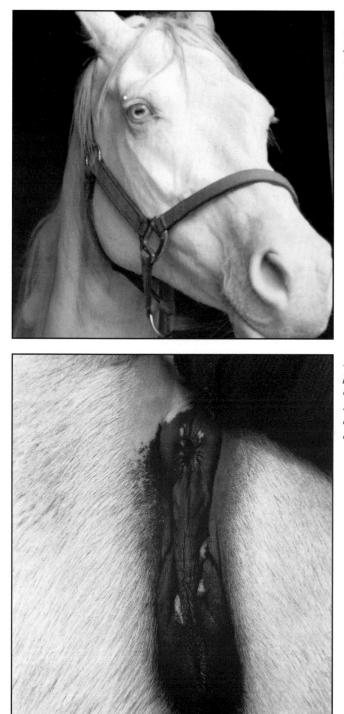

*This Palamino cross has no pigment in its skin or eyes – a cremello*

*Loss of skin pigment, as here on the perinaeum, sometimes follows equine coital exanthema*

*A temporary change of hair colour on* (right) *this horse's quarter resulted from a sweat mark due to a muscle tear*

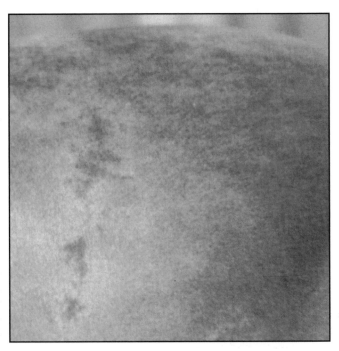

*The loss* (below) *of pigment in these hairs was due to firing with liquid nitrogen*

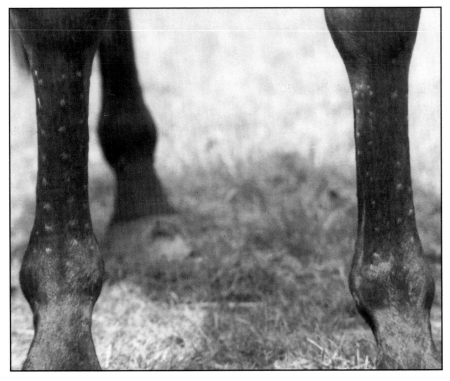

Leukotrichia is a condition seen in Thoroughbreds, Standardbreds and Quarterhorses in which small unpigmented areas of hair develop over the body of a previously normal animal. It follows temporary alopecia and is represented by white hairs that appear after a wound, or freeze-branding. Variegated or reticulated leukotrichia occurs in Standardbreds and Quarterhorses and is of unknown cause. In Thoroughbreds, leukotrichia can occur at any age though younger animals are most likely to be affected. It is not impossible that some of these white areas may disappear again in time.

Piebaldism is a congenital absence of pigment in areas of skin, with normal black pigmentation of others. It may be dominant or recessive in nature.

Strawberry birthmark (angiomatosis), consists of a hairless lesion seen on the extremities, consisting of a proliferation of blood vessels.

Vitiligo is a patchy loss of pigment in defined local areas. It is a tardive hereditary condition, a classical feature of Appaloosa pigmentation. It occurs as annular spots of depigmentation, seen on the muzzle and about the eyes, is commonly seen in Arabian horses and is sometimes not permanent. Vitiligo is caused by the breakdown of skin pigments and may be provoked by tack in certain situations. It can also occur as a consequence of other skin conditions such as auto-immune conditions. It is harmless and is similar to a condition that occurs in humans.

## Hormonal Diseases

Hirsutism (or excessive hairiness) is a condition of aged horses frequently related to tumours of the pituitary gland. The condition is associated with abnormally high levels of circulating cortisol and there is a possible link between the excessive hair growth and blood progesterone levels in affected animals.

Tumours of the adrenal gland might alternatively be implicated, as can protracted corticosteroid therapy.

As well as hirsutism, symptoms may include undue thirst or hunger, polyuria (excessive urination), sweating, weight loss and greater susceptibility to infection.

Diagnosis is made dependent on the symptoms. Blood and urine tests and skin biopsies will lead towards the same conclusion, although results are not normally specific.

While treatments, both medical and surgical, are a possiblity in pituitary tumours encountered in human practice, aesthetic considerations

*Hirsutism due to a
pituitary tumour*

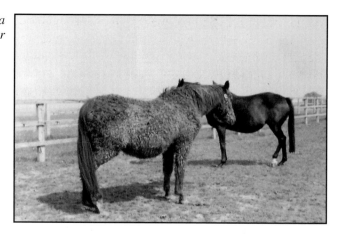

will prevail in dealing with horses. Among these are age, usefulness and, above all, value. Clearly, prolonging the life of a valuable stallion or mare will be considered important, although the possibility is that reduced fertility will go hand in hand with other symptoms.

## Hypothyroidism

Goiter, or enlarged thyroid glands (situated at the upper end of the jugular furrow at each side) is a feature of hypothyroidism.

Other symptoms include poor skin health with surface scaling and a broken mane. Affected animals may be lethargic and unable to peform effectively when trained. Broodmares may fail to produce milk and their foals may have deformed limbs.

Affected animals may prove to be anaemic, but skin biopsy tests are not specific in diagnosis. Blood tests can be carried out to evaluate thyroid hormone release although these have not all been fully evaluated for the horse and there are limitations.

Hormonal treatment is not necessarily effective and some horses with the above symptoms will respond favourably to the inclusion of an available source of iodine added to the diet.

## Immune Diseases

The normal functioning of the immune system involves the production of antibodies against foreign materials so that the body can rid itself of these materials when they are encountered again.

The most common way this happens relates to bacterial, viral and parasitic diseases, where exposure to infection results in the development of specific antibodies, a case in point being influenza, where the development of antibodies usually means an affected animal is resistant to infection by the same virus for an undefined period thereafter.

An undesireable by-product of this mechanism is the production of auto-antibodies against an animal's own tissues. This process is recognised in different animals and man and has recently been observed in the horse. Antibodies are produced against various body cells, including blood cells, and the abnormal activity of the immune system may be triggered by conditions like viral infections, but there may also be a genetic aspect to it.

The recognised signs of the condition, called lupus erythematosus, are joint enlargements, kidney disease, anaemia, oedema of the limbs and abdomen, skin disease and persistent fever that fails to respond to antibiotics. There may also be involvement of the respiratory system, and organs such as heart and muscle.

Skin abnormalities vary from excessive scaling to red areas, hair and pigment loss. Exposed mucous membranes in areas such as the mouth, nose, vulva and penis may show indications of ulcers. Alopecia, hair loss, and leukoderma (loss of pigmentation), are also seen.

Diagnosis of the condition is dependent on tests such as the antinuclear antibody test, and tissue biopsy.

Symptomatic treatment of the condition is the only possible response using anti-inflammatory drugs like corticosteroids and others which may help to suppress the immune system.

A less severe expression of the same condition is that of discoid lupus erythematosus in which there is hair and pigment loss, mostly of the head and neck without systemic signs. In this condition avoidance of intense sunlight is important and surface use of barrier or corticosteroid creams can be useful.

Another similar condition recorded in the horse, and one most common in Appaloosas, is pemphigus foliaceus (the term 'pemphigus' signifies blister in Greek). There is skin scaling and pustule development which may be restricted to the head and ears or become more generalised. Oedema, depression and fever may also occur.

Pemphigoid is a similar kind of condition in which lesions are confined to mucous membranes or to their junctions with the skin. Blisters in this case lead to ulceration.

The condition alopecia areata is sometimes seen in horses and is also considered to be immune-mediated. Circumscribed areas of hair loss are

*Skin lesions associated with* pemphigus foliaceus. *Note the skin is dry and scaling*

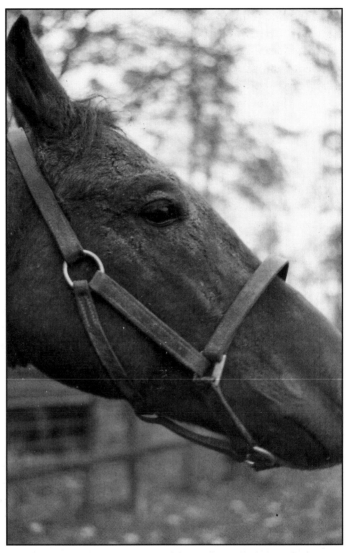

typical and the condition is diagnosed on the basis of cellular changes seen when examining biopsies microscopically.

Also thought to be immune-mediated, erythema multiforme occurs symmetrically and most frequently involves the limbs. Lesions appear as spots and blisters. Peripheral spread is common, leaving a radiating type of lesion. Treatment involves detection and elimination of underlying causes.

A condition in which skin lesions develop following infections such as *Streptococcus equi*, immune-mediated disorders, reactions to injection and their like, cutaneous vasculitis also occurs in horses frequently as a sequel to purpura haemorrhagica and is considered to be an immune-mediated disease. The principle lesion relates to changes within blood vessels of the skin, and occurs on dependent parts of the body, feet and ears; it has the appearance of an elevated bruise that may later regress leaving a hollow area where it previously existed.

# Keratinization Disorders

Keratinization disorders are conditions in which there is a problem with skin cell production; scaling, crusting, greasiness and hair loss are the primary signs. Self-trauma may lead to secondary infection from, for example, bacteria which results in a foul odour. Antiseborrhoeic shampoos may be used to cleanse the skin and then are rinsed off. Linear keratosis occurs in Quarter Horses, Morgans, Standardbreds, and Percherons. Lesions occur on the neck and lateral thorax showing hair loss and scaling in linear bands. There is some suggestion that the condition may arise as a result of larval migration. Cannon keratosis occurs on the hind cannons with scaling, crusting and hair loss.

# Lymphangitis

Lymphangitis is a condition of the lymphatic vessels that carry lymph into the veins (and liver) from the extremities. Along the course of lymphatic vessels, the lymph glands are set, their purpose to filter off foreign material, including organisms, and prevent these from getting deeper into the body.

The swelling in lymphangitis is extreme and usually only one limb is affected. The tissue inflammation involves the lymphatic vessels and glands. The whole leg may be swollen from the ground to stifle or elbow.

The term lymphangitis mainly applies to a condition marked by extensive filling of one hind leg. It occurs in housed animals on hard feeding most commonly. It may be precipitated by trauma or infection.

Swelling is gross and the limb may appear stretched to capacity. The skin may even weep in severe cases. There is usually localised pain on the course of leg vessels. The animal may sweat and have a raised temperature. Lameness of the affected limb is marked.

Diagnosis is based on the nature and size of the swelling and the condition must not be confused with physical injuries.

Antihistamine and anti-inflammatory drugs are used to control the tissue reactions which lead to the condition. In some cases the response is quick. Laxative diets and purgatives may help as may diuretics. It is important to encourage the animal to use the affected limb in order to assist circulation.

The affected limb may retain permanent signs after recovery and recurring episodes are common in individual cases; each of these may leave the leg a little larger. Horses which have suffered one attack should be regularly exercised and lightly lunged on rest days.

## Nodular Panniculitis

Nodular panniculitis is an inflammatory condition of subcutaneous fat, the cause of which is poorly understood. Lesions may be local or generalised and vary in size. They are sometimes painful and may ulcerate, causing marked scarring when lesions heal.

## Unilateral Papular Dermatosis

Unilateral papular dermatosis occurs on the neck and trunk and consists of bunches of intradermal papules which are most commonly seen

*Nodular lesions on the face and neck*

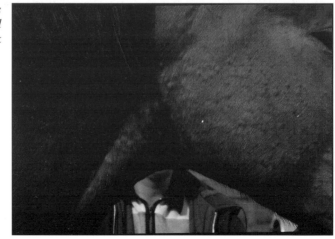

in Quarter Horses. The condition may be a sign of a hypersensitivity reaction.

## Poll Evil

Poll evil is a similar condition to fistulous withers occurring in the supra-atlantal bursa that underlies the ligamentum nuchae in the region of the poll, immediately behind the ears. It is an infectious condition, considered to be associated with the organism that causes brucellosis, and has become rare in modern times.

## Protozoan Skin Diseases

Leishmaniasis is a rare disease. It occurs mostly in Mediterranean countries and parts of the USA, is spread by sandflies (*Phlebotomus* among others) and also by blood transfusions. Rats, mice, dogs and cats are reservoir hosts. There may be localised skin lesions or systemic signs. Diagnosis is based on finding the organism microscopically within tissue scavanger cells. Because of an implied risk to public health, affected animals are usually humanely destroyed.

## Saddle Sores and Girth Galls

Saddle sores and girth galls are caused by pressure on areas tack

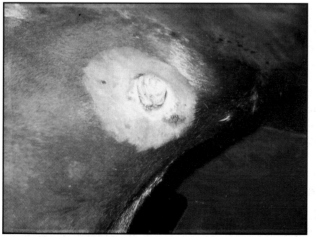

*Sitfast caused by a re-padded saddle*

comes in contact with. Saddle sores may be small and circumscribed or more extensive depending on the cause. Improperly fitting and badly sprung saddles tend to be a prime cause and sometimes poor riding techniques are to blame. Lesions are particularly tender where they overly bone.

Apart from local treatment, it is critical that affected areas be saved from further pressure if the horse is being ridden. This can be arranged by the use of foam padding and may be helped by numerous types of protection available through saddlers.

Therapeutic ultrasound or lasers are very useful for taking the aggravation out of this type of lesion, but it is always critical to prevent further aggravation by ensuring that the injured area does not come in contact with tack until fully healed.

# Viral Diseases

Equine coital exanthema (ECE) is a contagious venereal disease caused by the herpesvirus EHV3. Incubation is about seven days and transmission may occur by direct contact, by fomites, including surgical instruments, and through respiratory secretions.

The infection is expressed by papules, vesicles and pustules on the penis, prepuce and vulva. Lesions may also occur on the mouth, nose or lips. Areas lacking pigment may result after this infection.

Diagnosis is based on the signs and virus isolation may be successful in some cases.

The condition resolves spontaneously in one to two weeks and may be aided by the use of local antibiotic sprays to prevent secondary infection of healing lesions. Affected stallions should not be used until the infection has resolved, but mares may be bred from successfully on the next oestrus period. It is highly unusual to see a recurrence of this condition in an individual animal.

## Horse Pox

Horse pox is a rare, benign disease caused by vaccinia virus.

## Molluscum Contagiosum

Molluscum contagiosum is a mildly contagious infection of viral origin in which multiple greyish papules of a waxy consistency appear about the muzzle, perineum and other parts of the horse's body. It occurs in both sexes. The condition is self-limiting.

## Vesicular Stomatitis

Vesicular stomatitis is a viral disease that affects horses, cattle, swine and sometimes humans. There are vesicles on the lips and tongue and also on the coronary band where they may lead to hoof defects.

Treatment includes prevention of bacterial secondary infections. Recovery takes from one to five weeks.

## Equine Viral Arteritis

Equine viral arteritis (EVA) is a systemic highly infectious viral disease.

There are skin manifestations and subcutaneous oedema. Oedematous plaques occur on the side of the body, and there is oedema of the eyelids and legs. There may be scattered papules on the side of the face and neck, and urticarial type skin reactions over the trunk.

## Viral Papular Dermatitis

Viral papular dermatitis is a virus disease with an incubation period of about one week. Small papules appear in saddle and girth areas causing hair loss, crusting and local irritation for two to six weeks. Inevitably, fomites can be involved in the spread of an infection of this nature and good hygiene is important in prevention.

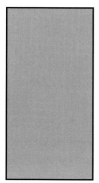

# Glossary

| | |
|---|---|
| abrasion | skin graze, as with rope burn, grazed knee |
| abscess | cavity filled with pus |
| acariasis | infestation with ticks or mites |
| acne | skin condition marked by pustules |
| albinism | inherited absence of pigment in hair, skin and eyes |
| allergen | substance capable of causing allergy |
| allergy | hypersensitivity to an antigen |
| allergic dermatitis | skin inflammation caused by allergy |
| allergic urticaria | hives, of allergic origin |
| alopecia | hair loss |
| alopecia areata | focal patches of alopecia |
| anaemia | lowered red blood cells and/or haemoglobin |
| aneurysm | dilatation of blood vessel wall |
| angioedema | condition marked by painless swellings under the skin and mucous membranes |
| anhidrosis | chronic dry coat |
| annular lesion | ring-shaped or circular lesion |
| antenna | head appendage of arthropod |
| antibiotic | chemical that inhibits or kills bacteria |
| antibody | body defence, produced by lymphocyte cells |
| antigen | causes antibody production (virus, bacterium, etc.) |
| antiseptic | inhibits or destroys organisms |
| aplasia cutis | hereditary absence of skin (as epitheliogenesis imperfecta) |
| arthropod | family that includes arachnids and insects |
| atheroma | cyst containing porridge-like exudate |
| aural plaque | ear lesion, raised and circumscribed, said to be form of papillomatosis |

| | |
|---|---|
| autoantibody | antibody against animal's own tissues |
| autogenous | derived from same animal; autogenous vaccine is produced from organisms taken from an affected animal |
| autoimmune | antibodies produced against own tissues |
| basal cell tumour | rare, benign tumour of skin |
| *Basidiobolus* | |
| *haptosporus* | cause of fungal skin disease |
| biopsy | sample from living tissue for diagnostic purposes |
| blowfly strike | invasion of skin by blowfly larvae |
| bulla | large blister |
| bullous | |
| pemphigoid | autoimmune skin disease |
| burn | tissue injury resulting from heat, cold, chemicals, etc. |
| bursa | fluid-filled sac often between bone and tendon/muscle (false bursa – forms on the knee, etc., as a result of injury; spinous bursitis – fistulous withers) |
| calcinosis | |
| circumscripta | localised nodule of calcium |
| callus | local thickening of skin due to friction, etc. |
| *Candida* | fungal organism that may be associated with disease |
| Canadian | |
| horsepox | pustular skin disease |
| cellulitis | inflammatory reaction spreading beneath the skin |
| cercaria | larval stage of liver fluke |
| *Cestoda* | class to which tapeworms belong |
| chemotherapy | treatment by chemical substances or drugs |
| *Coccidia* | protozoan cause of enteric disease |
| coital exanthema | viral venereal disease |
| colic | pain of abdominal origin |
| collagen | structural protein of white fibres of skin, etc. |
| complement | a body defensive substance |
| congenital | a mark or condition present at birth |
| *Conidiobolus* | |
| *coronatus* | fungal infection of nasal cavities. |
| crust | dried skin exudate |
| cryosurgery | surgery by freezing, either with dry ice (liquid nitrogen) or carbon dioxide |
| cutaneous | |
| habronemiasis | *see* habronemiasis |
| cutis | the skin |
| cytology | diagnostic examination of cells |
| decubital ulcer | skin ulcer due to lying down |
| depigmentation | loss of colour from skin |
| dermatology | study of skin disease |

| | |
|---|---|
| *Dermatophilus* | bacterial cause of rain scald and greasy heel |
| dermatophyte | organism that causes fungal infection of skin |
| dermis | skin area between epidermis and fat layers |
| dermoid cyst | hereditary lesion often seen on skin |
| dorsal shield | plate or scutum on hard ticks |
| eczema | inflammation of the outer skin layer |
| electrosurgery | surgery by use of an electric current |
| embolus | clot in blood, blocking artery (usually part of thrombus) |
| emollient | agent that soothes irritation |
| endocrinology | study of hormones |
| eosinophil | a type of white blood cell |
| eosinophilic granuloma | subcutaneous nodules containing eosinophils |
| epidermal collarette | circular epidermal lesion |
| epidermis | outer layer of skin |
| epitheliogenesis imperfecta | *see* aplasia cutis |
| erosion | a shallow surface skin lesion |
| erythema | redness of skin |
| erythema multiforme | immune complex disease with annular lesions |
| erythroderma | redness of skin over wide area |
| EVA | equine viral arteritis |
| excoriation | superficial graze, as from scratching |
| exfoliate | to shed |
| exfoliative dermatitis | increased skin scaling |
| exudate | discharge like pus or serum |
| fibroma | benign fibrous tissue tumour |
| fibrosarcoma | malignant fibrous tissue tumour |
| fissure | skin crack |
| fistula | open skin tract, possibly from deep infection |
| folliculitis | inflammation of hair follicles |
| fomes (fomites) | inanimate object capable of spreading infection |
| furunculosis | skin boils |
| gangrene | death of body tissue with invasion by saprophytic bacteria (dry gangrene occurs with arterial damage at peripheral sites, such as the ear; gas gangrene infection caused by anerobic organisms; moist gangrene caused by loss of blood supply, as in torsion) |
| granuloma | tumour-like mass of granulation tissue |
| guard hairs | long hairs of body coat |
| habronemiasis | disease caused by *Habronema* species (also called summer |

|  | sores, bursatii, swamp cancer, kunkers, esponja and granular dermatitis) |
| --- | --- |
| haematoma | subcutaneous swelling consisting of blood |
| haemangioma | benign tumour of blood vessels |
| helminth | parasitic worm |
| hereditary | genetically transmitted trait |
| hirsutism | hairy state |
| histology | microscopic study of tissue |
| histopathology | microscopic study of abnormal tissue |
| histoplasmosis | fungal infection with primary focus in lungs (also cause of epizootic lymphangitis, pseudoglanders or African farcy) |
| horsepox | a benign disease caused by a poxvirus. |
| hyperhydrosis | excessive sweating, often seen after prostaglandin injection |
| hyperkeratosis | hypertrophy of skin horny layer |
| hypertrichosis | hirsutism |
| hypodermis | subcutis |
| hypo-pigmentation | reduction in normal pigmentation |
| hypotrichosis | alopecia |
| hyper-pigmentation | increased skin pigmentation |
| immuno-pathology | study of immune diseases |
| immuno-therapy | therapy designed to aid or stimulate immunity |
| induration | hardening of skin |
| infection | disease caused by microorganisms or internal parasites |
| infestation | parasitic disease of the skin |
| inflammation | tissue reaction to insult or infection |
| *Insecta* | class of arthropods |
| intradermal | within the skin |
| ischaemic necrosis | local tissue loss on ears, etc., a symptom of ergot poisoning |
| keratin | protein of epidermis, etc. |
| larvicidal | kills larvae |
| leiomyosarcoma | malignant tumour of smooth muscle |
| lesion | pathological tissue |
| leukoderma | depigmentation after injury, etc. |
| leukotrichia | whitening of hair after injury |
| lichenification | thickening and folding of the skin |
| lipoma | a benign tumour of fat |
| lymphocyte | a white blood cell |
| lymphoedema | oedema due to lymphatic obstruction |
| lymphoma | tumour of lymphoid tissue |

| | |
|---|---|
| macrophage | scavenger cell of tissue |
| macule | skin spot |
| mange | disease caused by mites |
| mast cell | body defensive cell |
| mastocytoma | mast cell tumour |
| melanoma | tumour common in grey horses |
| melanosarcoma | malignant melanoma |
| metacercaria | larval stage of liver fluke |
| metastasis | spread of disease from one organ to another |
| microfilaria | larval stage of worms like *Onchocerca* and *Setaria* |
| *Microsporum* | fungus causing ringworm |
| miracidium | larval stage of liver fluke |
| molloscum contagiosum | skin disease caused by a poxvirus |
| monocyte | a white blood cell |
| mycetoma | subcutaneous bacterial or fungal growth |
| mycosis | disease caused by fungi |
| myiasis | body invasion by fly larvae |
| necrosis | process of cell death |
| *Nematoda* | roundworm class |
| neoplasia | growth formation |
| neoplasm | new growth, usually refers to tumour |
| neurofibroma | benign tumour of peripheral nerve |
| neutrophil | a white blood cell |
| nodule | solid lump of skin |
| nodular necrobiosis | multiple nodules of skin in horse |
| oedema | fluid accumulation under skin or in body cavity |
| otoscope | instrument for ear examination |
| panniculitis | inflammatory condition of subcutaneous fat |
| papillomatosis | refers to multiple wart growth |
| papule | small elevation of skin |
| parasite | organism that lives on another |
| paresis | partial paralysis, often of hind legs |
| patch | defined skin lesion |
| pemphigus foliaceus | general scaling disease |
| phaeohypomy- cosis | diffuse fungal dermatitis |
| photodermatitis | condition of skin due to sunlight exposure |
| photo- sensitisation | acquired reaction of skin to sunlight |
| plaque | large patch |
| polydypsia | abnormal thirst |

| | |
|---|---|
| polyphagia | abnormal hunger |
| polyuria | excessive urination |
| predilection site | situation parasite lives in/on body |
| proboscis | sucking mouthpart of insect |
| prognosis | likely disease outcome |
| *Protozoa* | single-cell family of organisms (includes *Coccidia*) |
| proud flesh | exuberant wound granulation |
| pruritis | itchiness |
| pustule | pimple filled with pus |
| pyoderma | purulent skin disease |
| redia | larval stage of liver fluke |
| reservoir host | animal that acts as source of infection for others, usually without showing signs of disease |
| resistance | ability to withstand disease, or drug |
| ringworm | a fungal infection of skin |
| sarcoid | skin tumour |
| scale | skin flake |
| scar | repaired (skin) after wound |
| schirrous cord | enlargement of spermatic cord after castration |
| sclerosis | hardening from inflammation |
| seborrhoea | increase of sebum production with scaling and crusts |
| sebum | oily product of sebaceous glands |
| sensitivity | open to disease, or organism susceptible to drug |
| serpiginous lesion | having wavy outline |
| serum | fluid part of blood after clotting |
| sinus | cavity, as in paranasal sinus, or open discharging tract |
| sitfast | sore on withers caused by saddle |
| sporotrichosis | fungal skin disease |
| squamous cell carcinoma | malignant tumour of skin/mucous membrane junction |
| St John's wort | a plant cause of photodermatitis |
| strangles | a bacterial disease marked by abscess formation |
| stratum | layer |
| stratum corneum | outer layer of the skin |
| subcutis | layer beneath the skin |
| subcutaneous emphysema | air or gas under skin |
| sweet itch | skin disease due to fly bites (also called Queensland itch, dhobie itch, Kasen, summer eczema) |
| sweat gland adenoma | benign tumour of sweat gland |
| tardive | late, inherited trait appearing after birth |
| tetanus | bacterial disease caused by *Clostridium tetani* |

| | |
|---|---|
| thermo-regulation | regulation of body temperature |
| thrombus | clot within vessel, may include worm larvae |
| titre | serum level measured against specific entity, like a virus |
| topical | application of drug, etc., to local skin area |
| toxin | a poison |
| *Trematoda* | parasitic family that includes fluke |
| *Trichophyton* | fungal cause of skin disease |
| trypanosomiasis | protozoan disease caused by *Trypanosoma* species |
| tumefaction | a skin swelling |
| tumour | a mass or swelling, synonymous with neoplasm |
| thermal injury | burn (including firing marks, cryosurgery) |
| ulcer | a lesion that penetrates the skin (or other tissues) |
| ulcerative lymphangitis | bacterial infection of lymphatics in lower limbs |
| unilateral papular dermatitis | papules that appear on one side only of horse, cause unknown |
| urticaria | hives |
| vellus hairs | smaller hairs of body coat |
| vesicle | small blister |
| vibrissae | sensory hairs or whiskers |
| vitiligo | local loss of skin pigment |
| wart | papilloma |
| wheal | urticarial lesion |
| zoonosis | disease transmitted from animal to man |
| zygomycosis | fungal skin disease |

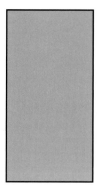

# Index